Thieme

Inflammation and Rheumatic Diseases

The molecular basis of novel therapies

Stefan Laufer, Steffen Gay, Kay Brune

With contributions by

Volker Bartsch
Fiorella Calanni
Renate E. Gay
Holm Häntzschel
Matthias Pierer
Ulf Wagner

42 Figures
23 Tables

Georg Thieme Verlag
Stuttgart · New York

Bibliographic Information published by
Die Deutsche Bibliothek

Die Deutsche Bibliothek lists this publication in the Deutsche Nationalbibliografie; detailled bibliographic data is available on the internet at http://dnb.ddb.de.

1., revised and updated English edition 2003
based on the 1. German edition 2002

Translated by Michael Capone
TR11 5UU Mawnan Smith, Great Britain

Rüdigerstraße 14
70469 Stuttgart, Germany
http://www.thieme.de
Thieme New York, 333 Seventh Avenue
New York, NY 10001, USA
http://www.thieme.com

Printed in Germany

Cover design by Thieme Verlagsgruppe
Cover photo: PhotoDisc, Inc.
Figures by Ziegler + Müller, Kirchentellinsfurt
Typesetting by Ziegler + Müller, Kirchentellinsfurt
Printing by Grammlich, Pliezhausen
Bookbinding by Held, Rottenburg

ISBN 3-13-133091-0 (GTV)
ISBN 1-58890-205-6 (TNY)

1 2 3 4 5 6

Important Note: Medicine is an ever-changing science undergoing continual development. Research and clinical experience are continually expanding our knowledge, in particular our knowledge of proper treatment and drug therapy. Insofar as this book mentions any dosage or application, readers may rest assured that the authors, editors, and publishers have made every effort to ensure that such references are in accordance with **the state of knowledge at the time of production of the book.**

Nevertheless, this does not involve, imply, or express any guarantee or responsibility on the part of the publishers in respect to any dosage instructions and forms of applications stated in the book. **Every user is requested to examine carefully** the manufacturers' leaflets accompanying each drug and to check, if necessary in consultation with a physician or specialist, whether the dosage schedules mentioned therein or the contraindications stated by the manufacturers differ from the statements made in the present book. Such examination is particularly important with drugs that are either rarely used or have been newly released on the market. Every dosage schedule or every form of application used is entirely at the user's own risk and responsibility. The authors and publishers request every user to report to the publishers any discrepancies or inaccuracies noticed.

Authors

Editors

Prof. Dr. rer. nat. Stefan Laufer
Eberhard-Karls-Universität
Pharmazeutisches Institut
Auf der Morgenstelle 8
72076 Tübingen

Prof. Dr. med. Steffen Gay
Director, WHO Collaborating Center
for Molecular Biology and Novel Therapeutic
Strategies for Rheumatic Diseases
Department of Rheumatology
University Hospital
Gloriastrasse 25
8091 Zürich
Schweiz

Prof. Dr. med. Dr. h.c. Kay Brune
Universität Erlangen-Nürnberg
Institut für Experimentelle
und Klinische Pharmakologie
Fahrstraße 17
91054 Erlangen

Contributors

Dr. med. Volker Bartsch
Am Stadtpfad 11
65760 Eschborn

Dr. rer. nat. Fiorella Calanni
Via Ragazzi del 99 n. 5
40133 Bologna
Italien

Prof. Dr. med. Renate E. Gay
Department of Rheumatology
University Hospital
Gloriastrasse 25
8091 Zürich
Schweiz

Prof. Dr. med. Holm Häntzschel
Zentrum für Innere Medizin
Universitätsklinikum Leipzig
Härtelstraße 16 – 18
04107 Leipzig

Dr. med. Matthias Pierer
Department of Rheumatology
University Hospital
Gloriastrasse 25
8091 Zürich
Schweiz

Dr. med. Ulf Wagner
Zentrum für Innere Medizin
Universitätsklinikum Leipzig
Härtelstraße 16 – 18
04107 Leipzig

Contents

1 Pathogenesis of Inflammatory Rheumatic Diseases of the Joints – Current Research Findings

Matthias Pierer, Ulf Wagner, Holm Häntzschel,
Renate E. Gay and Steffen Gay

1.1 Introduction

Inflammatory and degenerative diseases of the joints are common, affecting almost 50% of the population during the course of their lives. Rheumatoid arthritis (RA) is the most common of the inflammatory joint diseases, with a prevalence of 1%, and also has the most severe consequences for the patient. The destructive mechanisms involved in the advanced disease stage of RA bear similarities to other inflammatory joint diseases and, as a result, the recent molecular and cytological findings that have led to emerging concepts about the pathogenesis of RA are reviewed here.

In recent years, antibodies, receptor fusion proteins, and receptor antagonists blocking the cytokines tumor necrosis factor (TNF)-α and interleukin-1 have been successfully used in the treatment of RA and provide impressive examples of results from basic rheumatologic research [Feldmann et al., 1996]. The clinical success of these so-called biologicals highlights the key mediator function that these cytokines play in the inflammatory cascade. However, despite this success, only 50% of all patients who receive this treatment can expect to experience a significant improvement, and a still unknown proportion of patients experience a slowing or cessation of joint destruction. Clearly, inhibition of individual proinflammatory cytokines is not in itself sufficient to inhibit the activation of synovial tissue or stop the progress of joint destruction in most patients. These results also highlight the high degree of heterogeneity among RA patients. Hence, the concept of an independently acting cytokine network appears unlikely to be correct. Instead, a viewpoint now emerging is that both exogenous and endogenous factors play a significant role in this system. Many questions regarding the individual processes underlying the disease remain unanswered, and we are far from being able to formulate an overall concept that integrates all of the reported findings.

The identification of autoagglutinins or rheumatoid factors (later found to be autoantibodies to immunoglobulins), the detection of immune complexes in joints, and finally the discovery of polyclonal B-cell activation in the 1970s, led to the hypothesis that B cells are the major effectors of RA. Later, Stastny et al. found a correlation with specific human leukocyte antigen (HLA) alleles in RA and subsequently this was narrowed down to alleles possessing the so-called "shared epitope", a specific amino acid sequence (QKRAA) in the DR-β chain of the HLA class II molecule. For most researchers the identification of this sequence in the peptide-binding region of the HLA class II molecule was, in addition to a pathologic B-cell response, the pivotal argument for classifying RA as an autoimmune disease.

Nevertheless, even at the time, it was clear that 25% of RA patients do not possess the "shared epitope", while around 25% of healthy people are carriers. The actual function of the "shared epitope" remains unclear, although parallels from animal models would indicate a role in the presentation of specific arthritogenic antigens. This has been demonstrated in transgenic mice with human HLA-DR4. These mice selectively present the same collagen type II peptide as mice with the major histocompatibility complex (MHC) class II allele I-Aq; however, the latter increases the susceptibility of this mouse strain to collagen-induced arthritis [Fugger et al., 1996].

The relatively high percentage of $CD4^+$ T cells in the inflamed synovium, and the aforementioned HLA-DR association (HLA-DR molecules are the ligands of the T-cell receptor on CD4 T cells), have led to the view that RA is essentially a T-cell-mediated autoimmune disease. However, subsequent clinical studies targeting $CD4^+$ T cells achieved only limited success and, therefore, the role of these cells and indeed the role of the entire adaptive immune response in the chronic disease process have been questioned.

Hypothetically dividing the disease progress into the stages of initiation, destruction and perpetuation has proved useful for analyzing the pathophysiologic processes of rheumatoid synovitis. Molecular biological and cytological research in recent years has mainly helped to improve our understanding of the latter two stages of the disease process. The involvement of various immune and nonimmune cells, their communication via cytokines and cell interactions, and the processes leading to cartilage and bone destruction have been described in numerous papers, and many interesting therapeutic approaches are currently undergoing preclinical or clinical testing. Yet little is known about the actual triggering mechanisms – the etiology – which develops through a complex interplay of genetic and exogenous factors. The identity of the exogenous factors remains hidden, as neither viruses nor other infectious noxae have been confirmed. Moreover, the genetic factors, whose influence extends beyond the HLA system, (e.g. polymorphism of the TNF-α gene and prolactin

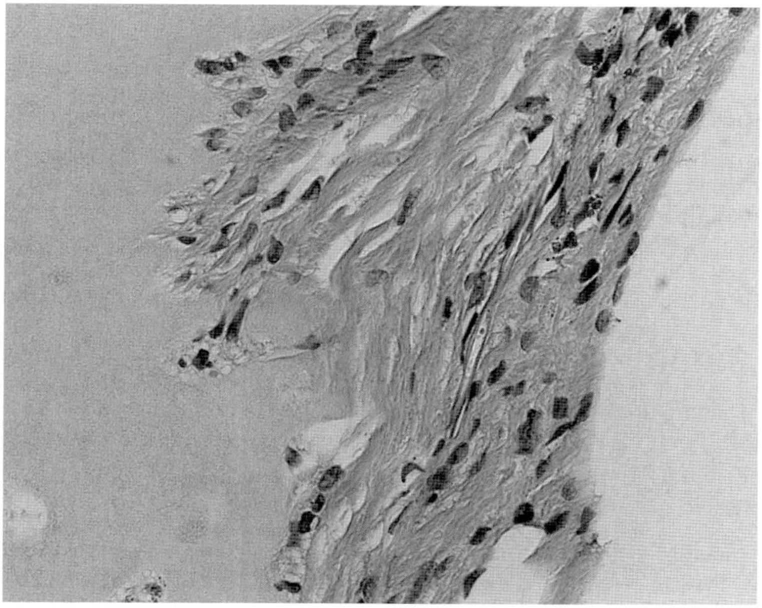

Fig. 1.**1** Invasion of rheumatoid arthritis fibroblasts (RA SF) into normal human cartilage engrafted into SCID mice. Independent of human inflammatory macrophages and T cells human RA SF invade into cartilage demonstrating an activated aggressively growing phenotype.

gene), have been described in contradictory terms.

After a decade-long search for malfunctions of individual cellular and molecular components, one viewpoint that is gaining popularity is that manifestation of the disease depends on a complex biological response of the innate and acquired immune systems combined with tissue-specific factors. It is hoped that the development of modern methods for characterizing these complex biological systems will improve our understanding of the pathogenesis of RA in the coming years.

At the center of RA pathology is the inflamed synovium. Synovial hyperplasia is characteristic of the disease and has been implicated in the associated destruction of joints [Kobayashi et al., 1975; Harris et al., 1970]. The synovium is a differentiated tissue exhibiting stage-typical and region-typical characteristics [Fassbender, 1983; Firestein, 1996; Müller-Ladner et al., 1997; Hamilton, 1983]. A striking and typical finding is thickening of the lining layer – the innermost layer of the synovium – from a single layer to as many as ten layers. These layers are no longer composed solely of resident synovial cells, but also contain numerous migratory cells. The majority are macrophages [Kelly et al., 1988; Burmester et al., 1997; Salisbury et al., 1987] and others exhibit typical features of fibroblasts. These cells, referred to as synovial fibroblasts (SFs), are mainly distinguished by the absence of the macrophage-specific markers CD68, CD11 b CD14 and CD33, and by the presence of small quantities of MHC class II molecules and the expression of prolyl-4-hydroxylase – an enzyme involved in collagen metabolism [Firestein, 1998 Hoyhtya et al., 1984]. Some of these cells have characteristics indicative of activation and are described as transformed-appearing or activated SFs [Firestein, 1996; Gay et al., 1993].

Marked changes also occur in the area consisting initially of loose connective tissue and in the deeper layers, known as the sublining. The infiltration of mononuclear cells, mainly T cells, macrophages, B cells, and plasma cells, occurs less uniformly in the sublining than in the lining layer [Ziff, 1989] (Fig. 1.**1**).

Approximately 20% of all biopsy specimens contain secondary aggregates of lymphatic infiltrates. Because of their follicle-like organization, these aggregates are reminiscent of lymph nodes with germinal centers [Wagner et al., 1998 b]. However, unlike the germinal centers of lymph nodes, the majority of cells within the CD4 T-cell population exhibit features of differentiation as memory cells with CD29/CD45RO expression [Ezawa et al., 1997; Matsuoka et al., 1991]. The ratio of CD4-positive to CD8-positive T cells within the sublining fluctuates from 4 : 1 to 14 : 1 [Meijer et al., 1982; Young et al., 1984]. This ratio is far higher than in either peripheral blood or synovial fluid [Firestein, 1998].

CD19-positive B lymphocytes also occur in this zone of inflamed synovium, often accumulating in clusters. Many of these B cells show signs of differentiation into plasma cells and are known to produce rheumatoid factors [Mellbye et al., 1990]. In producing rheumatoid factors and other autoantibodies, these B cells appear to be involved in the local inflammation process. Chronic inflammation evidently releases numerous antigens that are unable to induce negative selection in the thymus as they are not expressed as joint-specific antigens; secondary antibodies to these antigens are evidently produced, and these may play a role in the perpetuation of the disease process [Berek et al., 1997; De Clerck, 1995; Youinou et al., 1984].

The vascularization of the inflamed synovium differs from that of a healthy synovium in two respects. First, high-endothelial venules particularly favor the migration of lymphocytes [Girard and Springer, 1995]. Second, enhanced angiogenesis occurs. Although these changes are thought to be nonspecific and merely the consequence of inflammation, recent research indicates that they are responsible for the observed hyperplasia of the synovium [Koch, 1998].

A recently published study reported good success with specific antiangiogenetic treatment in an animal model of collagen-induced arthritis. By coupling a proapoptotic dimer heptapeptide to an RGD-containing peptide that recognizes endoluminally regulated integrin αVβ2 in inflamed tissue, it was possible to exert a positive influence on hyperplasia and inflammatory activity [Gerlag et al., 2001]. This highlights the important role played in the disease process by neovascularization and the vascular endothelium. The finding that concentrations of CD146 (which is produced almost exclusively by vascular endothelial cells) are elevated in the synovial fluid of patients with early RA lends further weight to this hypothesis [Neidhart et al., 1999].

Another characteristic feature of RA is the development of local invasive tissue known as a pannus. This tissue, which is located at sites of cartilage erosion, has been shown to be largely responsible for the destruction of joint cartilage and bone. "Pannus" differs histologically from other described regions of the synovium and shows phases of aggression. However, the term "pannus" has no scientific foundation as molecular markers used to characterize these cells reveal activation of various transcription factors and matrix-destroying enzymes. It appears, therefore, to be more appropriate to refer to the tissue as "activated" synovium.

Initially the tissue consists mainly of mononuclear cells and fibroblasts and produces large quantities of matrix metalloproteinases and cathepsins, especially in the cells of the lining layers [Shiozawa et al., 1983; Gravallese et al., 1991]. In later stages of the disease, the initially cell-rich tissue becomes increasingly fibrous until finally it consists of just a few blood vessels and a large proportion of collagen [Kobayashi and Ziff, 1975]. The origin of the cells in the activated synovium is not known, but many appear to be fibroblast-like synoviocytes. *In vitro* studies have shown that contact-inhibition of proliferation is impaired and the interactions of cells–cells and cells–matrix are modified – a typical feature of transformed cells [Lafyatis et al., 1989]. These aspects are dealt with in more detail in the section on the molecular mechanisms of joint destruction.

1.2 The major pathogenetic mechanisms of RA

The pathogenesis of RA involves migrated immune cells, such as T cells, B cells, plasma cells, macrophages, dendritic cells, neutrophils, granulocytes, and mast cells, as well as tissue-resident cells, such as synovial fibroblasts, chondrocytes, osteoblasts, and osteoclasts. All these cells act together in the inflamed synovium by communicating via soluble mediators (such as cytokines and chemokines) and by direct cell–cell contact mechanisms. The latter are more difficult to characterize. All the cells involved play various roles in the three main pathogenetic mechanisms of RA (Fig. 1.**2**).

Lymphoid cells in the pathogenesis of RA

T cells

As indicated earlier, there is considerable evidence that T cells play an active role in the pathogenesis of RA. T cells represent a large proportion of the mononuclear infiltrates in the sublining and may organize follicle-like cell structures in this region, similar to those present in lymph nodes and Payer's patches [Rooney et al., 1989].

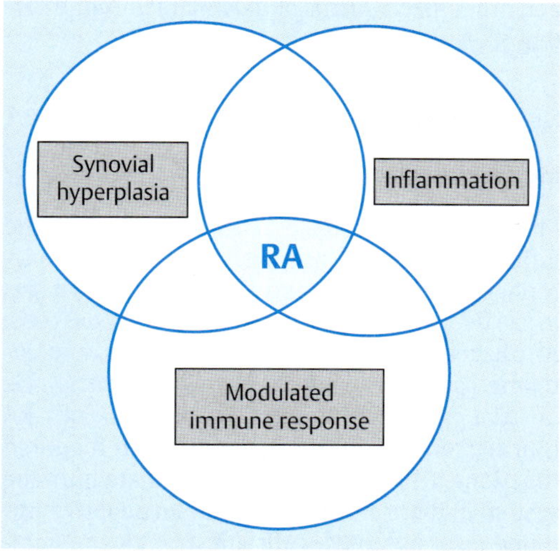

Fig. 1.2 Three major overlapping mechanisms are involved in the pathogenesis of joint destruction associated with RA [Gay et al., 1993].

Studies of the T-cell-receptor (TCR) repertoire within the synovium and peripheral blood have contributed significantly to our understanding of the function of T cells in RA. Although certain receptor sequences were found to be over-represented, most of the studies indicate the heterogeneous use of all receptor chains within the inflamed synovium – even if they appeared increased by cloning. This suggests the presence of a large number of T-cell antigens [Jenkins et al., 1993; Uematsu et al., 1991]. Other studies of peripheral T-cell homeostasis showed a limited TCR repertoire, specific changes in receptor selection, and clonal expansions, mainly in the CD4 cell compartment [Wagner et al., 1998 a]. These findings have given rise to one of the pathogenetic concepts of RA: aberrant systemic selection (thymic or peripheral) of T cells in conjunction with MHC class-II-mediated activation of these clonotypes in the joint. This explains the association with specific HLA alleles. The suspicion that the observed reduction in the TCR repertoire is a secondary phenomenon, due to the release of antigens during chronic inflammation, is opposed by the finding that the antigens are present even during the early stages of the disease. In addition, antigens have been shown to remain relatively constant in prospective studies [Schmidt et al., 1996]. However, little is known about the molecular causes of synovial inflammation arising from these conditions.

Despite numerous findings that suggest that T cells participate actively in the inflammatory process in joints, other findings indicate that T cells are not exclusively responsible for the activation of synovial cells in RA. Thus, research into the cellular kinetics of synovium-infiltrating T cells has demonstrated a low rate of proliferation [Nykanen et al., 1986]. Characterization of the CD45 isoforms on synovial T cells also revealed enrichment of markers typical of memory cells, in comparison to peripheral blood [Kohem et al., 1996; Koch et al., 1990]. This phenotype is more suggestive of recruitment of preactivated and mature T cells rather than *in situ* activation and maturation – for example by a range of joint-specific antigens. Finally, analysis of T cell cytokines in joints should be mentioned, as this found only small amounts of IL-2 and IL-2 R or interferon-γ. This observation contradicts the notion of a T-cell-mediated inflammatory process [Firestein et al., 1998]. Although the role of T cells in joint destruction has been challenged, they are clearly involved in both the systemic initiation and the perpetuation of RA.

B lymphocytes

Based on the development of a mouse model of spontaneous polyarthritis, by Mathis and Benoist, that has numerous parallels with the human disease, B lymphocytes experienced a renaissance in research. This was based on the observation that certain aspects of the disease can only be transmitted by serum or an immunoglobulin fraction and that the active component is an autoantibody to an ubiquitous enzyme involved in glycolysis [Matsumoto et al., 1999]. Although the extent to which this model reflects the real mechanisms of RA is disputed, B lymphocytes are an essential requirement for development of the disease. Analyses of the inflamed RA synovium also indicate the involvement of B lymphocytes.

Germinal centers are found in the synovium in 10–30% of RA patients [Takemura et al., 2001]. These contain B cells with V-region genes, suggesting clonal expansion and affinity maturation by somatic hypermutations [Gause et al., 1997]. Other studies into the V(D)J rearrangement of B cells from follicular regions have shown a gradual accumulation of somatic mutations during clonal expansion in synovial tissue. This clearly indicates a germinal-center reaction, which is otherwise found only in secondary lymphatic tissue. This finding favors the view that naive B cells migrate into the inflamed synovium causing local antigen-dependent activation [Kim et al., 1999].

For which cells are these B-cell receptor specific antigens? RA is characterized by the production of rheumatoid factors (RF)-autoantibodies to IgG found in the serum of most patients. B cells exhibiting such specificity have been isolated from various compartments including blood, bone marrow, synovial fluid, and synovium [Burastero et al., 1990; Ezaki et al., 1991; Krenn et al., 1999]. Rheumatoid factors could be responsible for, among other things, activating other B and T cells. It has been shown that RF-bearing B cells can bind immunoglobulin antigen complexes and, in so doing, internalize a number of different antigens [Roosnek and Lanzavecchia, 1991]. In this way, the processing and antigen presentation of peptides to T cells could lead to T-cell assistance and further activation of (auto)-antigen-specific B cells.

In recent years a number of other autoantibodies have been characterized, some with far greater specificity for RA than RF, although with less sensitivity. Researchers have identified a number of autoreactive intracytoplasmic antibodies to DNA: thyroglobulin [Randen et al., 1989], HLA-DR [Searles et al., 1988], heteronuclear ribonuclear protein A2 or RA33 [Hassfeld et al., 1989], calpastin [Yamamoto et al., 1992], antinuclear antibodies, and antineutrophil cytoplasmic antibodies (ANCA) [Mulder et al., 1993], calreticulin [Routsias et al., 1993], Sa antigen [Despres et al., 1994], p205 [Hain et al., 1996], filaggrin [Simon et al., 1993], glucose-6-phosphate-isomerase [Schaller et al., 2001], RASFp1 heptapeptide [von Landenberg et al., 1999], and endoplasmic reticulum chaperone protein (BiP) [Corrigall et al., 2001]. These antigens have been shown not only to induce autoantibodies, but also to elicit T-cell reactivity. As none of these antigens exhibit joint-specific expression, their direct contribution to the pathogenesis of articular destruction remains unknown. Moreover, as these antigens occur intracellularly, the question arises as to whether these antibodies are actually able to reach their antigens *in vivo*, and if this occurs what the consequences would be. However, the ubiquitous GPI antigen – the target antigen in the transgenic K/RxN mouse model – has recently been shown to be deposited on cartilage surfaces in the form of immune complexes, as in an Arthus reaction, leading to joint pathology by alternative activation of the complement cascade and other mechanisms of the innate immune system [Ji et al., 2002].

Nonlymphoid cells in the pathogenesis of RA

Monocytes/macrophages

Monocytes/macrophages occur at two sites in the inflamed synovium: as type A synoviocytes, macrophages of the lining layer, and as macrophages in the deeper layers accompanied by T and B cells. As phagocytes, antigen-presenting cells, and cytokine-producers, these cells play a central role in the pathophysiologic processes of RA [Burmester et al., 1997]. In view of their manifold functions, which form part of the innate immune system and are also essential for an adaptive immune response, these cells are strongly implicated in the pathogenesis of RA. As producers of the cytokines TNF-α and interleukin (IL)-1, their function can be inhibited by specific drugs, even though these cytokines are also synthesized by fibroblasts and T cells [Burmester et al., 1997]. Both cytokines are placed at the top of the cascade of inflammatory mediators, with TNF-α having a certain superiority, both induce the production of other cytokines, chemokines, or prostaglandins as well as metalloproteases and cathepsins. In addition, IL-1 has negative effects on the integrity of joints. It inhibits the synthesis of proteoglycans and induces matrix metalloproteinases (MMP) in chondrocytes [van-de Loof et al., 1995]. Immunohistological investigations of macrophages have established a direct correlation between the number of macrophages and joint destruction [Mulherin et al., 1996 a; Yanni et al., 1994]. Together with Fc-γ receptors and complement receptors, macrophages are potential mediators of pathological autoantibodies in the inflamed synovium. Investigations of Fc receptors on monocytes have shown that activation results mainly from Fc-γ III receptors [Abrahams et al., 2000], whereas Fc-γ II receptors have a counter-regulatory function, as demonstrated in a study using Fc-γ receptor II knock-out mice [Yuasa et al., 1999].

The accumulation of macrophages, which migrate out of the bloodstream as monocytes incapable of further division, appears due to an increased rate of transmigration of these cells into high endothelial venules, and the predestined synovial inhibition of apoptosis. Perlman and coworkers recently demonstrated apoptosis resistance to anti-Fas antibodies in synovial macrophages, as had previously been described for synovial RA fibroblasts, due to upregulation of the caspase inhibitor known as FLIP [Perlman et al., 2001]. Finally, it has been shown that synovial RA fibroblasts produce factors, like osteopontin, that attract macrophages [Petrow et al., 2000].

Synovial fibroblasts

The first observations that mesenchymal cells of the synovium, termed synovial fibroblasts (SFs), play a key role in the pathogenesis of RA were made in the late 1970s. Fassbender and coworkers found marked morphological differences between the cells in RA and those in osteoarthritis [Fassbender, 1983]. Recent years have seen much effort to characterize these fibroblasts, which Fassbender described as "transformed", at the functional, and molecular level.

Two notable animal models for investigating these cells have been developed: the MRL-lpr/lpr mouse and the severe, combined immuno-deficiency disease (SCID) mouse model of RA. MRL-lpr/lpr mice develop, in addition to other autoimmune phenomena, RF-positive erosive arthritis that bears many similarities to RA [O'Sullivan et al., 1985]. Using this model, it was shown that initial joint destruction is mediated by activated synovial cells [Tanaka et al., 1988]. Destruction in this model occurred only in regions in which direct adhesion of synoviocytes to cartilage and bone occurred.

Using the same model, Trabandt and coworkers demonstrated the constitutive expression of MMP-1 (matrix metalloproteinase-1, also called collagenase) in synoviocytes. Immunohistochemically, this degrading enzyme occurred predominantly in proliferating cells of the synovial lining and in chondrocytes [Trabandt et al., 1992 b]. Interestingly, these cells contained a high concentration of RNA for the proto-oncogene, c-fos. It was also observed in this model that inflammatory cells do not migrate into the synovium until cartilage destruction has already started, but then act to intensify the process. Antibody reactivity in the form of autoimmunity to collagen type II also developed only as a consequence of cartilage destruction. This finding challenges the paradigm of a primacy of inflammatory processes in RA-associated joint destruction [Kraan et al., 1998].

The co-implantation model of the SCID mouse, as a model of cartilage destruction mediated by human synovial fibroblasts, has found increasing use in recent years. Based on the results of Mosier and coworkers, who showed for the first time that a functional human immune system can be implanted into SCID mice, Rendt and coworkers implanted human RA synovium into these mice below the renal capsule [Mosier et al., 1988; Rendt et al., 1993]. This model, which was originally intended for investigating co-infused T cells, revealed a gradual disappearance of the human T cells from the engrafted synovium, while the synoviocytes not only survived, but retained their phenotype and functional characteristics.

From this, Geiler and coworkers developed the SCID mouse model of joint destruction which made it possible to examine new aspects of the molecular mechanisms underlying rheumatoid joint destruction [Geiler et al., 1994]. RA synovium was co-implanted in the SCID mice below the renal capsule together with normal human cartilage. The implanted synovial tissue, which was examined over a period of up to 200 days, exhibited the same invasive behavior as in human joints. The observation that the cells at the front of the invasion were mainly fibroblasts prompted us to use this model to investigate isolated RA fibroblasts and cartilage. It was found that the cartilage was gradually invaded and eroded just like intact RA synovial tissue [Müller-Ladner et al., 1996].

Comparison of these activated fibroblasts with fibroblasts from patients with osteoarthritis, which do not exhibit invasiveness in this model, suggests an aggressive phenotype of these cells in RA. This appears to correspond to the transformed phenotype described earlier by Fassbender [Müller-Ladner et al., 1996]. A decisive characteristic of cartilage-invading fibroblasts derived from patients with RA was the expression of cartilage-degrading proteases. In contrast, these proteases were expressed to only a small degree or not at all by fibroblasts from healthy skin and joints of patients with osteoarthritis.

Clinical observations and more recent studies have indicated a partial dissociation of joint inflammation and destruction, though the evidence is not entirely consistent. In this context, observations of RA patients with HIV infection need to be mentioned. Following HIV infection, a dramatic improvement in the clinical parameters of inflammation was observed and although the joints were not symptomatic the process of joint destruction continued unabated [Müller-Ladner et al., 1995 a]. A study by Mulherin and coworkers described the same phenomenon in 40 patients in whom erosive joint destruction progressed despite significant improvements in clinical and laboratory parameters of inflammation [Mulherin et al., 1996 b].

The pivotal mechanism of activation of synovial fibroblasts in the process of cartilage and bone destruction in RA is based on cytokine-dependent activation, impaired apoptosis, and the production of matrix-degrading enzymes (Fig. 1.**3**). The immediate cause of this aberrant behavior is still unknown. Proto-oncogenes and highly up-regulated transcription factors have been described in this context, suggesting a transformed-appearing phenotype (overview in Müller-Ladner et al., 1995 b).

A number of proto-oncogenes, including ras, raf, sis, myb, and myc, are up-regulated in RA tissues, especially in fibroblasts adhering to cartilage and bone. Recent findings indicate that some of these proto-oncogenes are directly involved in the upregulation of MMPs. The same applies to MMP-2 and MMP-9, which are regulated by growth hormones via the ras proto-oncogene [Gum et al., 1997; Korzus et al., 1997]. Although the cause of such proto-oncogene expression is unclear, it appears to result from specific signal cascades culminating in, among other mechanisms, the expression of MMPs.

Transcription factor activator protein (AP)-1, consisting of the elements c-fos and c-jun, is notably responsible for the production of matrix metalloproteinases and, therefore, for joint destruction in RA. c-fos, which is overexpressed in the synovium of RA patients [Trabandt et al., 1992a; Dooley et al., 1996], has a number of binding sites in the promoter region of specific MMP genes. Activity of AP-1, which can be measured by its ability to bind to the corresponding DNA sequence, was found mainly in adherent cells and correlated with clinical disease activity. However, the AP-1 binding sites in the promoter regions of the MMP genes were not the only enhancing regions [Asahara et al., 1997; Benbow and Brinckerhoff, 1997]. NFκB, the "inflammation transcription factor", is also strongly activated in synovial fibroblasts in RA [Miagkov et al., 1998]. As the target of proinflammatory cytokines, its activation leads further to the synthesis of proinflammatory cytokines as well as adhesion molecules and MMP [Vincenti et al., 1998]. A recently published study found marked inhibition of inflammation resulting from the gene transfer of IκBβ, a natural inhibitor of NFκB [Makarov et al., 1997]. The contribution of NFκB to joint destruction remains to be elucidated.

Because of their high rate of expression, transcription factor Wnt-5 A and its ligand, frizzled 5 (Fz5), which are involved in the differentiation of bone marrow stem cell precursors, have also been investigated as possible causes of the activated phenotype of synovial fibroblasts. After blockade by antisense RNA and in double-negative mutants, a significant reduction in the synthesis of IL-6 and IL-15 cytokines was found, supporting further the contribution of synovial fibroblasts to the inflammatory process [Sen et al., 2001].

In this context, tumor suppressor genes should also be mentioned. In recent years attention has focussed on these genes as a possible cause of the activated phenotype of synovial RA fibroblasts. Thus, it was shown that the tumor suppressor PTEN is not or only minimally expressed in the synovial lining layer in comparison to healthy synovium [Pap et al., 1998] In cultures, only 40 % of synovial RA fibroblasts express PTEN, and in the co-implantation model of the SCID mouse the aggressive cartilage-invading synovial cells specifically lack PTEN. In 1997 Firestein and coworkers discovered in the fibroblasts from RA patients somatic mutations of the tumor suppressor gene p53, similar to certain tumors [Firestein et al., 1997]. However, these findings have not been observed in other countries [Kullmann et al., 1999].

Another characteristic of synovial RA fibroblasts that is closely related to the aforementioned mechanisms is that of impaired apoptosis. In conjunction with an unchanged rate of proliferation (approximately 1 – 5 %), this disturbance contributes to the hyperplasia of the synovium. The current view of the development of synovial hyperplasia is not only based on the influx of monocytes, but also on the inhibition of apoptosis. In addition to evidence of disturbed sensitivity of the synovial cells to apoptosis induction by FasL [Nakajima et al., 1995], it has recently been shown that the antiapoptotic molecule sentrin is strongly expressed in RA synovial tissue [Franz et al., 1998 a] and may contribute to apoptosis resistance. The production of sentrin, which was up to 30 times more abundant *in vitro* than in control fibroblasts from osteoarthritis patients, was particularly expressed in the cells of the lining layer and the sites of joint destruction. bcl-2, which like sentrin possesses antiapoptotic activity, was also found but less abundantly in synovial

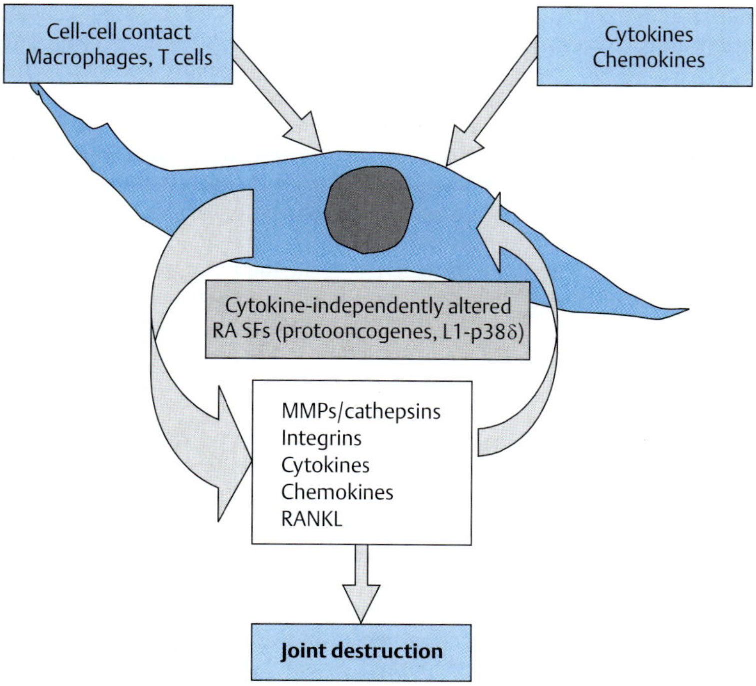

Fig. 1.3 Pathological functions of synovial fibroblasts in RA.

fibroblasts of the lining layer [Matsumoto et al., 1996].

On balance, the data support a preponderance of antiapoptotic versus proapoptotic signal paths, especially in synoviocytes of the lining layer. This imbalance may help to explain the prolonged life-span of activated fibroblasts mediating joint destruction.

Another exciting hypothesis regarding the origin of the aggressive behavior of RA SFs postulates independent activation of the cells by endogenous retroviral gene sequences and in turn the activation of other specific genes. Visualization of type C retroviral particles in the synovial fluid of RA patients by electron microscopy has, for the first time, lent support to this hypothesis [Stransky et al., 1993]. Further searches for endogenous retroviral RNA in the synovial fluid of RA patients revealed a large number of such sequences. The sequences also occur in healthy individuals, but RA is characterized by a typical expression pattern.

Retrotransposon L1, a residue of a former retrovirus that is distributed throughout the genome and represents an endogenous retroviral sequence lacking the coded segment for the capsid protein, was detected in RA SFs [Neidhart et al., 2000]. This led to a number of other interesting findings. Human L1 elements code for a protein approximately 40 kDa in size (ORF1/p40) which was found at sites of joint destruction Analyses of L1-p40/ORF1-transfected RA SFs revealed the induction of the stress-activated protein kinase p38 delta (SAPK2delta), which was also identified by immunohistology in RA SFs that aggressively invade joint structures [Neidhardt et al., 2000]. In addition to the aforementioned characteristics, which relate to the destructive potential of RA SFs, these cells are also important as producers of lymphocyte-activating cytokines. IL-15, expressed by RA SFs, attracts CD4-positive T cells, induces their proliferation, and inhibits their apoptosis [McInnes et al., 1996].

IL-16 must be mentioned in the same context. It is also produced by RA SFs and acts as a chemoattractant for CD4-positive T cells [Franz et al., 1998]. However, it exerts also opposite effects on these cells. It induces MHC class II molecules and the expression of IL-2 receptor [Center et al., 1996] described as activation markers. At the same time it energizes T cells [Theodore et al., 1996], a functional state that has been observed in articular T cells. RA SFs are, therefore, also decisively involved in the primarily antigen-independent migration, accumulation, and activation of T cells into joints in RA.

Osteoclasts

At the eroded zones of the bone, directly at the boundary between aggressive synovial tissue and bone, synovial fibroblasts, multinuclear osteoclasts, or both can usually be observed. The role of osteoclasts has been well described: they directly degrade bone [Gravallese et al., 1998]; without their help bone would probably not be attacked, as shown by recent data from animal models [Pettit et al., 2001].

However, the differentiation and activation of osteoclasts requires the help of other cells. In an animal model, either T cells or synovial RA fibroblasts were required to facilitate differentiation of these cells via expression of the receptor activator of the NFκB ligand (RANKL) [Lacey et al., 1998; Gravallese et al., 2000]. Osteoclasts are derived from myelomonocytic precursor cells, which are probably related to mesenchymal stem cells [Mbalaviele et al., 1999]. But precursor cells present in peripheral blood may also develop into osteoclasts *in vitro* after about 3 weeks [Zvaifler et al., 2000].

Osteoclasts also occur in RA tissue separate from erosion zones, often together with macrophages and cells bearing specific receptors for what are referred to as bone morphogenetic proteins [Marinova-Mutafchieva et al., 2000]. However, recent studies have shown that RA SFs contribute to osteoclast differentiation. Thus it has been demonstrated *in vitro* that RA SFs induce the differentiation of peripheral mononuclear blood cells to TRAP-positive multinuclear cells at a rate proportional to their synthesis of RANKL (osteoclast differentiation factor – ODF) [Shigeyama et al., 2000].

1.3 Summary

Despite the numerous findings that describe and explain the complex mechanisms operating in the pathogenesis of RA, the question regarding what triggers the disease remains unanswered. Whether the onset of the disease is characterized by an autoimmune process or by activation of nonspecific inflammatory mechanisms is a matter of speculation. The picture becomes clearer in the subsequent stage, which is characterized by inflammation. In this stage the main cellular players are macrophages, T cells, B cells, and synovial fibroblasts. This phase also marks the origin of T- and B-lymphocyte reactivity to neoantigens formed by the degradation of matrix components or nonspecifically in response to a chronic inflammatory milieu, resulting in intensification and prolongation of the inflammatory process.

Destruction of the joint structures begins during an early phase in which the clinical picture is dominated by inflammatory exudation with cartilage degradation and erosion. Bone degradation depends on the action of mature osteoclasts, which differentiate under the influence of synovial fibroblasts and T cells. Cartilage degradation, on the other hand, depends on the synthesis of proteolytic enzymes, which are released predominantly by synovial fibroblasts and granulocytes of the joint fluid. In later phases of the disease there is increasing dissociation of the inflammatory processes and further progress of joint destruction, which in the earlier phases may have been masked by cytokines such as TNF-α. This process is due chiefly to synovial RA fibroblasts characterized by an activated phenotype. This situation is due to the inflammatory milieu – mainly cytokines. However, there is much evidence in support of a cytokine-independent activation, e.g. activation due to endogenous retroviral sequences. Today's therapeutic methods provide no means for targeting these cells.

Future therapeutic methods that block strategic components of this network will ultimately help to elucidate their importance and permit stage-adapted treatment.

1.4 References

Abrahams VM, Cambridge G, Lydyard PM Edwards JC. Induction of tumor necrosis factor alpha production by adhered human monocytes: a key role for Fc gamma receptor type IIIa in rheumatoid arthritis. Arthritis Rheum 2000; 43: 608–616

Asahara H, Fujisawa K, Kobata T et al. Direct evidence of high DNA binding activity of transcription factor AP-1 in rheumatoid arthritis synovium. Arthritis Rheum 1997; 40: 912–918

Benbow U, Brinckerhoff CE. The AP-1 site and MMP gene regulation: what is all the fuss about? Matrix Biol 1997; 15: 519–526

Berek C, Kim HJ. B-cell activation and development within chronically inflamed synovium in rheumatoid and reactive arthritis. Semin Immunol 1997; 9: 261–268

Burastero SE, Cutolo M, Dessi V, Celada F. Monoreactive and polyreactive rheumatoid factors produced by in vitro Epstein–Barr virus-transformed peripheral blood and synovial B lymphocytes from rheumatoid arthritis patients. Scand J Immunol 1990; 32: 347–357

Burmester GR, Stuhlmuller B, Keyszer G, Kinne RW. Mononuclear phagocytes and rheumatoid synovitis. Mastermind or workhorse in arthritis? Arthritis Rheum 1997; 40: 5–18

Center DM, Kornfeld H, Cruikshank WW. Interleukin 16 and its function as a CD4 ligand. Immunol Today 1996; 17: 476–481

Corrigall VM, Bodman-Smith MD, Fife MS et al. The human endoplasmic reticulum molecular chaperone BiP is an autoantigen for rheumatoid arthritis and prevents the induction of experimental arthritis. J Immunol 2001; 166: 1492–1498

De Clerck LS. B lymphocytes and humoral immune responses in rheumatoid arthritis. Clin Rheumatol 1995; 14 (Suppl 2): 14–18

Despres N, Boire G, Lopez-Longo FJ, Menard HA. The Sa system: a novel antigen-antibody system specific for rheumatoid arthritis. J Rheumatol 1994; 21: 1027–1033

Dooley S, Herlitzka I, Hanselmann R et al. Constitutive expression of c-fos and c-jun, overexpression of ets-2, and reduced expression of metastasis suppressor gene nm23-H1 in rheumatoid arthritis. Ann Rheum Dis 1996; 55: 298–304

Ezaki I, Kanda H, Sakai K et al. Restricted diversity of the variable region nucleotide sequences of the heavy and light chains of a human rheumatoid factor. Arthritis Rheum 1991; 34: 343–350

Ezawa K, Yamamura M, Matsui H, Ota Z, Makino H. Comparative analysis of CD45RA- and CD45RO-positive CD4 + T cells in peripheral blood, synovial fluid, and synovial tissue in patients with rheumatoid arthritis and osteoarthritis. Acta Med Okayama 1997; 51: 25–31

Fassbender HG. Histomorphological basis of articular cartilage destruction in rheumatoid arthritis. Coll Relat Res 1983; 3: 141–155

Feldmann M, Brennan FM, Maini RN. Role of cytokines in rheumatoid arthritis. Annu Rev Immunol 1996; 14: 397–440

Firestein GS. Invasive fibroblast-like synoviocytes in rheumatoid arthritis. Passive responders or transformed aggressors? Arthritis Rheum 1996; 39: 1781–1790

Firestein GS. Rheumatoid synovitis and pannus. In: Klippel JH, Dieppe PA (eds). Rheumatology. London: Mosby, 1998: 5.13.1–5.13.24

Firestein GS, Echeverri F, Yeo M, Zvaifler NJ, Green DR. Somatic mutations in the p53 tumor suppressor gene in rheumatoid arthritis synovium. Proc Natl Acad Sci USA 1997; 94: 895–900

Franz JK, Hummel KM, Aicher WK et al. Invasive synovial fibroblasts express the novel anti-apoptotic molecule sentrin in the SCID mouse model of rheumatoid arthritis. Arthritis Rheum 1998 a; 41: S238

Franz JK, Kolb SA, Hummel KM et al. Interleukin-16, produced by synovial fibroblasts, mediates chemoattraction for CD4 + T lymphocytes in rheumatoid arthritis. Eur J Immunol 1998 b; 28: 2661–2671

Fugger L, Rothbard JB, Sonderstrup-McDevitt G. Specificity of an HLA-DRB1*0401-restricted T cell response to type II collagen. Eur J Immunol 1996; 26: 928–933

Gause A, Gundlach K, Carbon G et al. Analysis of VH gene rearrangements from synovial B cells of patients with rheumatoid arthritis reveals infiltration of the synovial membrane by memory B cells. Rheumatol Int 1997; 17: 145–150

Gay S, Gay RE, Koopman WJ. Molecular and cellular mechanisms of joint destruction in rheumatoid arthritis: two cellular mechanisms explain joint destruction? Ann Rheum Dis 1993; 52 (Suppl 1): S39–S47

Geiler T, Kriegsmann J, Keyszer GM, Gay RE, Gay S. A new model for rheumatoid arthritis generated by engraftment of rheumatoid synovial tissue and normal human cartilage into SCID mice. Arthritis Rheum 1994; 37: 1664–1671

Gerlag DM, Borges E, Tak PP et al. Suppression of murine collagen-induced arthritis by targeted apoptosis of synovial neovasculature. Arthritis Res 2001; 3: 357–361

Girard JP, Springer TA. High endothelial venules (HEVs): specialized endothelium for lymphocyte migration. Immunol Today 1995; 16: 449–457

Gravallese EM, Darling JM, Ladd AL, Katz JN, Glimcher LH. In situ hybridization studies of stromelysin and collagenase messenger RNA expression in rheumatoid synovium. Arthritis Rheum 1991; 34: 1076–1084

Gravallese EM, Harada Y, Wang J-T et al. Identification of cell types responsible for bone resorption in rheumatoid arthritis and juvenile rheumatoid arthritis. Am J Pathol 1998; 152: 943–951

Gravallese EM, Manning C, Tsay A et al. Synovial tissue in rheumatoid arthritis is a source of osteoclast differentiation factor. Arthritis Rheum 2000; 43: 250–258

Gum R, Wang H, Lengyel E, Juarez J, Boyd D. Regulation of 92 kDa type IV collagenase expression by the jun aminoterminal kinase- and the extracellular signal-regulated kinase-dependent signaling cascades. Oncogene 1997; 14: 1481–1493

Hain NA, Stuhlmuller B, Hahn GR et al. Biochemical characterization and microsequencing of a 205-kDa synovial protein stimulatory for T cells and reactive with rheumatoid factor containing sera. J Immunol 1996; 157: 1773–1780

Hamilton JA. Hypothesis: in vitro evidence for the invasive and tumor-like properties of the rheumatoid pannus. J Rheumatol 1983; 10: 845–851

Harris ED, DiBona DR, Krane SM. A mechanism for cartilage destruction in rheumatoid arthritis. Trans Assoc Am Physicians 1970; 83: 267 – 276

Hassfeld W, Steiner G, Hartmuth K et al. Demonstration of a new antinuclear antibody (anti-RA33) that is highly specific for rheumatoid arthritis. Arthritis Rheum 1989; 32: 1515 – 1520

Hoyhtya M, Myllyla R, Piuva J, Kivirikko KI, Tryggvason K. Monoclonal antibodies to human prolyl 4-hydroxylase. Eur J Biochem 1984; 141: 472 – 482

Jenkins RN, Nikaein A, Zimmermann A, Meek K, Lipsky PE. T cell receptor V beta gene bias in rheumatoid arthritis. J Clin Invest 1993; 92: 2688 – 2701

Ji H, Ohmura K, Mahmood U et al. Arthritis critically dependent on innate immune system players. Immunity 2002; 16: 157 – 168

Kelly PM, Bliss E, Morton JA, Burns J, McGee JO. Monoclonal antibody EBM/11: high cellular specificity for human macrophages. J Clin Pathol 1988; 41: 510 – 515

Kim HJ, Krenn V, Steinhauser G, Berek C. Plasma cell development in synovial germinal centers in patients with rheumatoid and reactive arthritis. J Immunol 1999; 162: 3053 – 3062

Kobayashi I, Ziff M. Electron microscopic studies of the cartilage–pannus junction in rheumatoid arthritis. Arthritis Rheum 1975; 18: 475 – 483

Koch AE. Review: angiogenesis: implications for rheumatoid arthritis. Arthritis Rheum 1998; 41: 951 – 962

Koch AE, Robinson PG, Radosevich JA, Pope RM. Distribution of CD45RA and CD45RO T-lymphocyte subsets in rheumatoid arthritis synovial tissue. J Clin Immunol 1990; 10: 192 – 199

Kohem CL, Brezinschek RI, Wisbey H et al. Enrichment of differentiated CD45RBdim, CD27-memory T cells in the peripheral blood, synovial fluid, and synovial tissue of patients with rheumatoid arthritis. Arthritis Rheum 1996; 39: 844 – 854

Korzus E, Nagase H, Rydell R, Travis J. The mitogen-activated protein kinase and JAK-STAT signaling pathways are required for an oncostatin M-responsive element-mediated activation of matrix metalloproteinase 1 gene expression. J Biol Chem 1997; 272: 1188 – 1196

Kraan MC, Versendaal H, Jonker M et al. Asymptomatic synovitis precedes clinically manifest arthritis. Arthritis Rheum 1998; 41: 1481 – 1488

Krenn V, Konig A, Hensel F et al. Molecular analysis of rheumatoid factor (RF)-negative B cell hybridomas from rheumatoid synovial tissue: evidence for an antigen-induced stimulation with selection of high mutated IgVH and low mutated IgVL/lambda genes. Clin Exp Immunol 1999; 115: 168 – 175

Kullmann F, Judex M, Neudecker I et al. Analysis of the p53 tumor suppressor gene in rheumatoid arthritis synovial fibroblasts. Arthritis Rheum 1999; 42: 1594 – 1600

Lacey DL, Timms E, Tan H-L et al. Osteoprotegerin ligand is a cytokine that regulates osteoclast differentiation and activation. Cell 1998; 93: 165 – 176

Lafyatis R, Remmers EF, Roberts AB et al. Anchorage-independent growth of synoviocytes from arthritic and normal joints: stimulation by exogenous platelet-derived growth factor and inhibition by transforming growth factor-beta and retinoids. J Clin Invest 1989; 83: 1267 – 1276

Makarov SS, Johnston WN, Olsen JC et al NF-kappaB as a target for anti-inflammatory gene therapy: suppression of inflammatory responses in monocytic and stromal cells by stable gene transfer of I kappa B alpha cDNA. Gene Ther 1997; 4: 846 – 852

Marinova-Mutafchieva L, Taylor P, Funa K, Maini RN, Zvaifler NJ. Mesenchymal cells expressing bone morphogenetic protein receptors are present in the rheumatoid arthritis joint. Arthritis Rheum 2000; 43: 2046 – 2055

Matsumoto S, Müller-Ladner U, Gay RE, Nishioka K, Gay S. Ultrastructural demonstration of apoptosis, Fas and Bcl-2 expression of rheumatoid synovial fibroblasts. J Rheumatol 1996; 23: 1345 – 1352

Matsumoto I, Staub A, Benoist C, Mathis D. Arthritis provoked by linked T and B cell recognition of a glycolytic enzyme. Science 1999; 286: 1732 – 1735

Matsuoka N, Eguchi K, Kawakami A et al. Phenotypic characteristics of T cells interacted with synovial cells. J Rheumatol 1991; 18: 1137 – 1142

Mbalaviele G, Jaiswal N, Meng A et al. Human mesenchymal stem cells promote human osteoclast differentiation from CD34 + bone marrow hematopoietic progenitors. Endocrinology 1999; 140: 3736 – 3743

McInnes IB, al-Mughales J, Field M et al. The role of interleukin-15 in T-cell migration and activation in rheumatoid arthritis. Nat Med 1996 2: 175 – 182

Meijer CJ, de Graaff-Reitsma CB, Lafeber GJ, Cats A. In situ localization of lymphocyte subsets in synovial membranes of patients with rheumatoid arthritis with monoclonal antibodies. J Rheumatol 1982; 9: 359 – 365

Mellbye OJ, Vartdal F, Pahle J, Mollnes TE. IgG and IgA subclass distribution of total immunoglobulin and rheumatoid factors in rheumatoid tissue plasma cells. Scand J Rheumatol 1990; 19: 333 – 340

Miagkov AV, Kovalenko DV, Brown CE et al. NF-kappaB activation provides the potential link between inflammation and hyperplasia in the arthritic joint. Proc Natl Acad Sci USA 1998; 95: 13859 – 13864

Mosier DE, Gulizia RJ, Baird SM, Wilson DB. Transfer of a functional human immune system to mice with severe combined immunodeficiency. Nature 1988; 335: 256 – 259

Mulder AH, Horst G, van Leeuwen MA, Limburg PC, Kallenberg CG. Antineutrophil cytoplasmic antibodies in rheumatoid arthritis. Characterization and clinical correlations. Arthritis Rheum 1993; 36: 1054 – 1060

Mulherin D, Fitzgerald O, Bresnihan B. Synovial tissue macrophage populations and articular damage in rheumatoid arthritis. Arthritis Rheum 1996 a; 39: 115–124

Mulherin D, Fitzgerald O, Bresnihan B. Clinical improvement and radiological deterioration in rheumatoid arthritis: evidence that the pathogenesis of synovial inflammation and articular erosion may differ. Br J Rheumatol 1996 b; 35: 1263–1268

Müller-Ladner U, Kriegsmann J, Gay RE et al. Progressive joint destruction in a human immunodeficiency virus-infected patient with rheumatoid arthritis. Arthritis Rheum 1995 a; 38: 1328–1332

Müller-Ladner U, Kriegsmann J, Gay RE, Gay S. Oncogenes in rheumatoid synovium. Rheum Dis Clin North Am 1995 b; 21: 675–690

Müller-Ladner U, Kriegsmann J, Franklin BN et al. Synovial fibroblasts of patients with rheumatoid arthritis attach to and invade normal human cartilage when engrafted into SCID mice. Am J Pathol 1996; 149: 1607–1615

Müller-Ladner U, Gay RE, Gay S. Cellular pathways of joint destruction. Curr Opin Rheumatol 1997; 9: 213–220

Nakajima T, Aono H, Hasunuma T et al. Apoptosis and functional Fas antigen in rheumatoid arthritis synoviocytes. Arthritis Rheum 1995; 38: 485–491

Neidhart M, Rethage J, Kuchen S et al. Retrotransposable L1 elements expressed in rheumatoid arthritis synovial tissue: association with genomic DNA hypomethylation and influence on gene expression. Arthritis Rheum 2000; 43: 2634–2647

Neidhart M, Wehrli R, Brühlmann P et al. Synovial fluid CD146 (MUC18), a marker for synovial membrane angiogenesis in rheumatoid arthritis. Arthritis Rheum 1999; 42: 622–630

Nykanen P, Bergroth V, Raunio P, Nordstrom D, Konttinen YT. Phenotypic characterization of ^{3}H-thymidine incorporating cells in rheumatoid arthritis synovial membrane. Rheumatol Int 1986; 6: 269–271

O'Sullivan FX, Fassbender HG, Gay S, Koopman WJ. Etiopathogenesis of the rheumatoid arthritis-like disease in MRL/l mice. I. The histomorphologic basis of joint destruction. Arthritis Rheum 1985; 28: 529–536

Pap T, Hummel KM, Franz JK et al. Downregulation but no mutation of novel tumor suppressor PTEN in aggressively invading rheumatoid arthritis fibroblasts (RA-SF). Arthritis Rheum 1998; 41: S239

Perlman H, Pagliari LJ, Liu H et al. Rheumatoid arthritis synovial macrophages express the Fas-associated death domain-like interleukin-1, beta-converting enzyme-inhibitory protein and are refractory to Fas-mediated apoptosis. Arthritis Rheum 2001; 44: 21–30

Petrow PK, Hummel KM, Schedel J et al. Expression of osteopontin messenger RNA and protein in rheumatoid arthritis: effects of osteopontin on the release of collagenase 1 from articular chondrocytes and synovial fibroblasts. Arthritis Rheum 2000; 43: 1597–1605

Pettit AR, Ji H, von Stechow D et al. TRANCE/RANKL knockout mice are protected from bone erosion in a serum transfer model of arthritis. Am J Pathol 2001; 159: 1689–1699

Randen I, Thompson KM, Natvig JB, Forre O, Waalen K. Human monoclonal rheumatoid factors derived from the polyclonal repertoire of rheumatoid synovial tissue: production and characterization. Clin Exp Immunol 1989; 78: 13–18

Rendt KE, Barry TS, Jones DM et al. Engraftment of human synovium into severe combined immune deficient mice. Migration of human peripheral blood T cells to engrafted human synovium and to mouse lymph nodes. J Immunol 1993; 151: 7324–7336

Roosnek E, Lanzavecchia A. Efficient and selective presentation of antigen–antibody complexes by rheumatoid factor B cells. J Exp Med 1991; 173: 487–489

Rooney M, Whelan A, Feighery C, Bresnihan B. The immunohistologic features of synovitis, disease activity and in vitro IgM rheumatoid factor synthesis by blood mononuclear cells in rheumatoid arthritis. J Rheumatol 1989; 16: 459–467

Routsias JG, Tzioufas AG, Sakarellos-Daitsiotis M, Sakarellos C, Moutsopoulos HM. Calreticulin synthetic peptide analogues: anti-peptide antibodies in autoimmune rheumatic diseases. Clin Exp Immunol 1993; 91: 437–441

Salisbury AK, Duke O, Poulter LW. Macrophage-like cells of the pannus area in rheumatoid arthritic joints. Scand J Rheumatol 1987; 16: 263–272

Schaller M, Burton DR, Ditzel HJ. Autoantibodies to GPI in rheumatoid arthritis: linkage between an animal model and human disease. Nat Immunol 2001; 2: 746–753

Schmidt D, Goronzy JJ, Weyand CM. CD4 + CD7– CD28– T cells are expanded in rheumatoid arthritis and are characterized by autoreactivity. J Clin Invest 1996; 97: 2027–2037

Searles RP, Savage SM, Brozek CM, Marnell LL, Hoffman CL. Network regulation in rheumatoid arthritis. Studies of DR+ T cells, anti-DR, antiidiotypic antibodies, and clinical disease activity. Arthritis Rheum 1988; 31: 834–843

Sen M, Chamorro M, Reifert J, Corr M, Carson DA. Blockade of Wnt-5 A/frizzled 5 signaling inhibits rheumatoid synoviocyte activation. Arthritis Rheum 2001; 44: 772–781

Shigeyama Y, Pap T, Kunzler P et al. Expression of osteoclast differentiation factor in rheumatoid arthritis Arthritis Rheum 2000; 43: 2523–2530

Shiozawa S, Shiozawa K, Fujita T. Morphologic observations in the early phase of the cartilage–pannus junction: light and electron microscopic studies of active cellular pannus. Arthritis Rheum 1983; 26 472–478

Stansky P. Association of the B-cell alloantigen DRw4 with rheumatoid arthritis. N Engl J Med 1978, 298 869–871

Simon M, Girbal E, Sebbag M et al. The cytokeratin filament-aggregating protein filaggrin is the target of the so-called "antikeratin antibodies", autoantibodies specific for rheumatoid arthritis. J Clin Invest 1993; 92: 1387–1393

Stransky G, Vernon J, Aicher WK et al. Virus-like particles in synovial fluids from patients with rheumatoid arthritis. Br J Rheumatol 1993; 32: 1044–1048

Takemura S, Braun A, Crowson C et al. Lymphoid neogenesis in rheumatoid synovitis. J Immunol 2001; 167: 1072–1080

Tanaka A, O'Sullivan FX, Koopman WJ, Gay S. Etiopathogenesis of rheumatoid arthritis-like disease in MRL/1 mice: II. Ultrastructural basis of joint destruction. J Rheumatol 1988; 15: 10–16

Theodore AC, Center DM, Nicoll J et al. CD4 ligand IL-16 inhibits the mixed lymphocyte reaction. J Immunol 1996; 157: 1958–1964

Trabandt A, Aicher WK, Gay RE et al. Spontaneous expression of immediately-early response genes c-fos and egr-1 in collagenase-producing rheumatoid synovial fibroblasts. Rheumatol Int 1992 a; 12: 53–59

Trabandt A, Gay RE, Birkedal Hansen H, Gay S. Expression of collagenase and potential transcriptional factors in the MRL/l mouse arthropathy. Semin Arthritis Rheum 1992 b; 21: 246–251

Uematsu Y, Wege H, Straus A et al. The T-cell-receptor repertoire in the synovial fluid of a patient with rheumatoid arthritis is polyclonal. Proc Natl Acad Sci USA 1991: 88: 8534–8538

van-de Loof FA, Joosten LA, van Lent P, Arntz OJ, van-den Berg BW. Role of interleukin-1, tumor necrosis factor alpha, and interleukin-6 in cartilage proteoglycan metabolism and destruction. Effect of in situ blocking in murine antigen- and zymosan-induced arthritis. Arthritis Rheum 1995; 38: 164–172

Vincenti MP, Coon CI, Brinckerhoff CE. Nuclear factor kappaB/p50 activates an element in the distal matrix metalloproteinase 1 promoter in interleukin-1 beta-stimulated synovial fibroblasts. Arthritis Rheum 1998; 41: 1987–1994

von Landenberg P, von Landenberg C, Grundl M et al. A new antigenic epitope localized within human kappa light chains specific for rheumatoid arthritis and systemic lupus erythematosus. J Autoimmun 1999; 13: 83–87

Wagner UG, Koetz K, Weyand CM, Goronzy JJ. Perturbation of the T cell repertoire in rheumatoid arthritis. Proc Natl Acad Sci USA 1998 a; 95: 447–452

Wagner UG, Kurtin PJ, Wahner A et al. The role of CD8 + CD40 L+ T cells in the formation of germinal centers in rheumatoid synovitis. J Immunol 1998 b; 161: 6390–6397

Yamamoto S, Shimizu K, Shimizu K et al. Calcium-dependent cysteine proteinase (calpain) in human arthritic synovial joints. Arthritis Rheum 1992; 35: 1309–1317

Yanni G, Whelan A, Feighery C, Bresnihan B. Synovial tissue macrophages and joint erosion in rheumatoid arthritis. Ann Rheum Dis 1994; 53: 39–44

Youinou PY, Irving WL, Shipley M, Hayes J, Lydyard PM. Evidence for B cell activation in patients with active rheumatoid arthritis. Clin Exp Immunol 1984; 55: 91–98

Young CL, Adamson TC, Vaughan JH, Fox RI. Immunohistologic characterization of synovial membrane lymphocytes in rheumatoid arthritis. Arthritis Rheum 1984; 27: 32–39

Yuasa T, Kubo S, Yoshino T et al. Deletion of fcgamma receptor IIB renders H-2(b) mice susceptible to collagen-induced arthritis. J Exp Med 1999; 189: 187–194

Ziff M. Pathways of mononuclear cell infiltration in rheumatoid synovitis. Rheumatol Int 1989; 9: 97–103

Zvaifler NJ, Marinova-Mutafchieva L, Adams G et al. Mesenchymal precursor cells in the circulation of normal individuals. Arthritis Res 2000; 2: 477–488

2 Biochemistry and Mediators of Inflammation

Fiorella Calanni, Stefan Laufer

2.1 Introduction

Inflammation is one of the most important, complex, and dynamic processes involved in the defense of the organism. It is initiated in response to tissue injury or infection. The inflammatory response involves a sequential release of many chemical mediators, which generate a multiplicity of vascular and cellular reactions. Of these, no other autacoids have such numerous and dissimilar physiologic effects as the prostanoids. These chemical mediators have not only a broad spectrum of activity but also a diverse range of quantitative and qualitative activities.

The family of autacoids known as prostanoids, which include the prostaglandins, prostacyclin, thromboxanes, and the leukotrienes, are derived from 20-carbon essential fatty acids that contain three, four or five double bonds, e.g. arachidonic acid (AA). In humans AA is the predominant precursor. It is either derived from dietary linoleic acid or ingested as a dietary constituent. It is then esterified to the phospholipids of cell membranes or other complex lipids. In view of the fact that the intracellular concentration of free arachidonate is very low, the biosynthesis of prostanoids depends primarily upon the availability of arachidonate to prostanoid-synthesizing enzymes. This results from its release from cellular stores of lipids by acylhydolases, most notably phospholipase A_2. Once released from the phospholipids of cell membranes, AA can be further metabolized by several enzymatic complexes, such as cyclooxygenases (COX) and lipoxygenases (LOX). In the cyclooxygenase pathways AA is transformed by specific synthases into thromboxane A_2 (TXA_2), prostacyclin (PGI_2), and prostaglandins (PGs). In the lipoxygenases pathways it is converted to leukotrienes (LTs) and lipoxins (LXs).

This work will focus on a detailed description of the metabolic pathways of arachidonic acid, as those enzymatic activities generate metabolites which act as mediators of many important facets of the inflammatory process and other physiologic and pathologic events. It will also discuss the mechanism of action, side effects, and clinical implications of the nonselective and selective COX-2 inhibitors and the combined inhibition of the two enzymes by lipoxygenase/cyclooxygenase inhibitors.

2.2 Phospholipase A_2

Phospholipase A_2 (PLA_2) comprises a class of enzymes that catalyze the hydrolysis of membrane phospholipids to release free fatty acids. The existence of these enzymes has been known for over 100 years [1], but it is only within the past 20 years that their importance in the biological processes has been appreciated [2].

PLA_2 activated in response to various physiologic stimuli cleaves the *sn*-2-acyl bond of phospholipids, particularly phosphatidylcholine and phosphatidylethanolamine, releasing, in equimolar quantities, lysophospholipids and free essential fatty acids, especially AA, the most abundant polyunsaturated fatty acid in the phospholipid component of cell membranes [2]. Once activated, PLA_2 can mediate a variety of pathophysiologic reactions, either through direct action or through subsequent transformation of its products (lysophospholipids and AA) to form several potent biologically active substances, such as prostaglandins, thromboxanes (TXs), leukotrienes, and platelet-activating factor (PAF) [2] (see Fig. 2.**1**). Acetylation of lysophospholipids at the 2-hydroxy group therefore gives rise to the lipid mediator PAF, a potent platelet-aggregating substance and inducer of various inflammatory reactions, such as erythema, chemotaxis, and increased vascular permeability [2]. Prostaglandins, thromboxanes, and leukotrienes, products formed from cyclooxygenase and 5-lipoxygenase-catalysed AA transformation, complete the family of inflammatory and allergic mediators derived from PLA_2 activation [2].

PLA_2 is a superfamily of enzymes that are widespread, being found in nearly all cell types [2].

In mammals, two isoforms of PLA_2 have been identified which do not share sequence homology and differ in their catalytic mechanism and regulation: a secretory PLA_2 ($sPLA_2$) and an intracellular PLA_2 [3] (see Fig. 2.**2**).

Secretory PLA_2 are enzymes of relatively low molecular weight and require millimolar concentrations of Ca^{++} for their activity. They are the principal enzymes responsible for the liberation of AA from membrane phospholipids in response to inflammatory stimuli and are therefore referred to collectively as the "inflammatory enzyme". They play a pre-eminent role in pathologic processes following inflammatory phenomena [4–6].

Intracellular PLA_2 are enzymes of high molecular weight and require micromolar or no con-

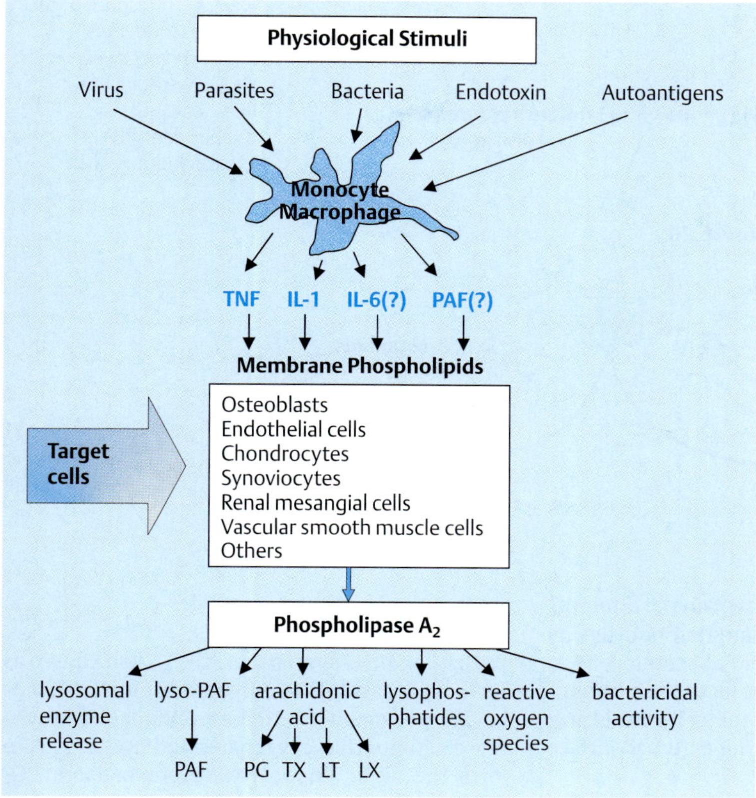

Fig. 2.**1** PLA_2 activation in response to various physiological stimuli. IL: interleukine; TNF: tumor necrosis factor; PAF: platelet-activating factor; PG: prostaglandin's; Tx: thromboxanes; LT: leukotrienes; LX: lipoxins.

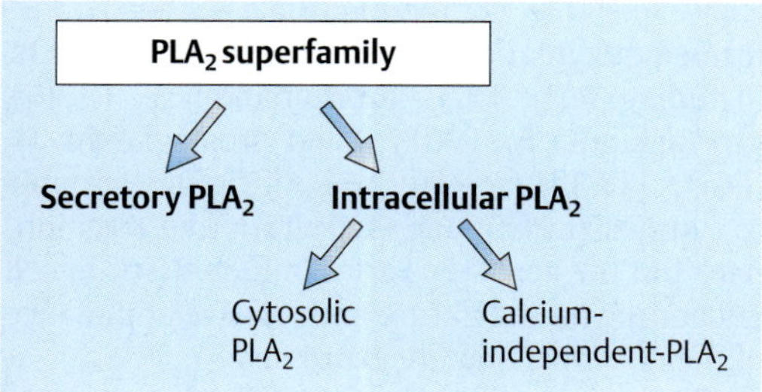

Fig. 2.**2** Isoforms of phospholipase A_2.

centrations of Ca^{++}. They include two types of enzyme: cytosolic phospholipase A_2 ($cPLA_2$), which is specific for AA-containing phospholipids and is therefore considered important in the liberation of AA and thus in the production of prostanoids, and calcium-independent phospholipase A_2 ($iPLA_2$), which is mainly involved in maintenance of the membrane phospholipid composition [4–6].

Under basal conditions and prior to stimulation $iPLA_2$ is the predominant phospholipase that hydrolyzes membrane phospholipids, liberating quantities of AA too small for conversion to prostanoids which are then recycled by the action of acyclases to reform membrane phospholipids [7] (Fig. 2.**3**). Following receptor activation, Ca^{++} levels rise, and inducible $cPLA_2$ becomes the predominant phospholipase involved in the release of free AA in sufficient quantities to be metabolized by specific enzymes to form prostanoids [7] (Fig. 2.**3**). After prolonged receptor occupancy and activation, the secretory form ($sPLA_2$) is induced. This enzyme is secreted and can therefore activate prostanoid synthesis in neighboring cells via a paracrine mechanism [7] (Fig. 2.**3**).

Apart from generating the most important lipid mediators of inflammation by binding to their own receptors, PLA_2 themselves produce vasoconstriction and bronchospasm and encourage the development of tumors and the invasiveness of tumor cells. Their action on membrane phospholipids is greatly enhanced by the presence of free radicals [8–11].

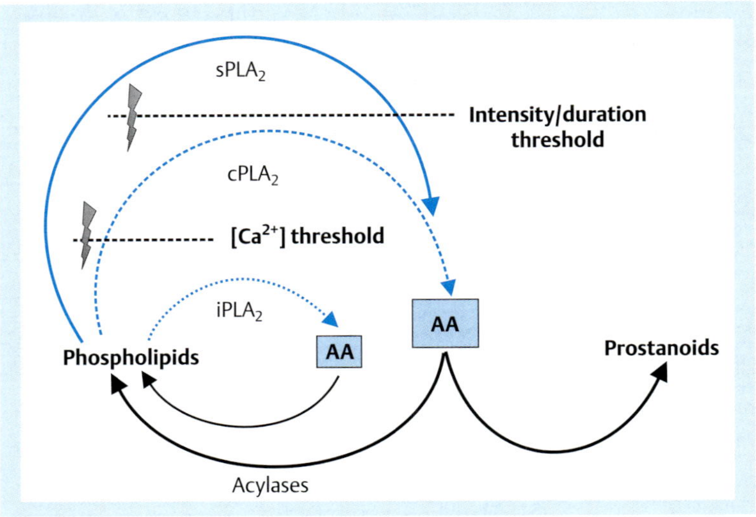

Fig. 2.**3** Phospholipase A_2 isoforms induction. $SPLA_2$: secretory PLA_2; $cPLA_2$: cytosolic PLA_2; $iPLA_2$: calcium-independent PLA_2; AA: arachidonic acid.

The above considerations explain the attempts to obtain innovative anti-inflammatory drugs by developing selective inhibitors of secretory PLA_2 [12]. Interest has particularly focused on inhibitors that are unable to cross the cell membrane, as these can act on $sPLA_2$ in the external surface of the membrane.

2.3 Arachidonic acid cascade

Prostanoids, derived from the precursor AA, are involved in a variety of clinically important areas such as inflammation, fever, thrombosis, allergic and immune responses, and cancer. They are produced by a variety of cell-type, tissue, and species-specific biosynthetic pathways. The prostanoid family (see Fig. 2.**4**) encompasses thromboxanes (TXs), PGs, LTs, hydroxyeicosatetraenoic acids (HETEs), epoxyeicosatrienoic acids (EETs), LXs, and isoprostanes, the latter of which can be generated by a nonenzymatic oxidative mechanism and may serve as markers of oxidative stress in humans. Each class of enzymatically produced prostanoids governs a specific set of functions and serves as mediator or autacoid acting within a local microenvironment to orchestrate key cellular responses.

The classical enzymes that metabolize AA to oxygenated products are:
- Cyclooxygenases (COX)
- Lipoxygenases (LOX)

Cyclooxygenases

Prostaglandin H synthases (PGHS), also known as cyclooxygenases (COX), are microsomal enzymes having two distinct activities: endoperoxide synthase activity that oxygenates and cyclizes AA to form the cyclic endoperoxide prostaglandin G_2 (PGG_2), and peroxidase activity that converts PGG_2 to prostaglandin H_2 (PGH_2). PGH_2 is a chemically unstable compound that is then transformed enzymatically into a variety of products, including PGI_2, TXA_2, prostaglandin E_2 (PGE_2), prostaglandin $F_{2\alpha}$ ($PGF_{2\alpha}$), and prostaglandin D_2 (PGD_2) [13, 14] (see Fig. 2.**5**). All tissues are able to synthesize PGG_2 and PGH_2 from free arachidonate, but the next step varies in each tissue or cell depending on the nature and relative abundance of the enzymes that are expressed.

The preferred substrates of COX contain at least three double bonds in a well-defined position. In addition to AA, these are dihomogammalinolenic acid and eicosapentenoic acid (EPA), which have three and five double bonds, respectively. COX can oxygenate other fatty acids lacking the three double bonds in the required positions to hydroperoxy fatty acids but not to PGs.

Structure of COX-1 and COX-2

In mammalian cells, COX exists in at least two isoforms: cyclooxygenase-1 (COX-1) and cyclooxygenase-2 (COX-2) [15 – 17]. COX-1 and COX-2 isoforms are structurally distinct proteins, with

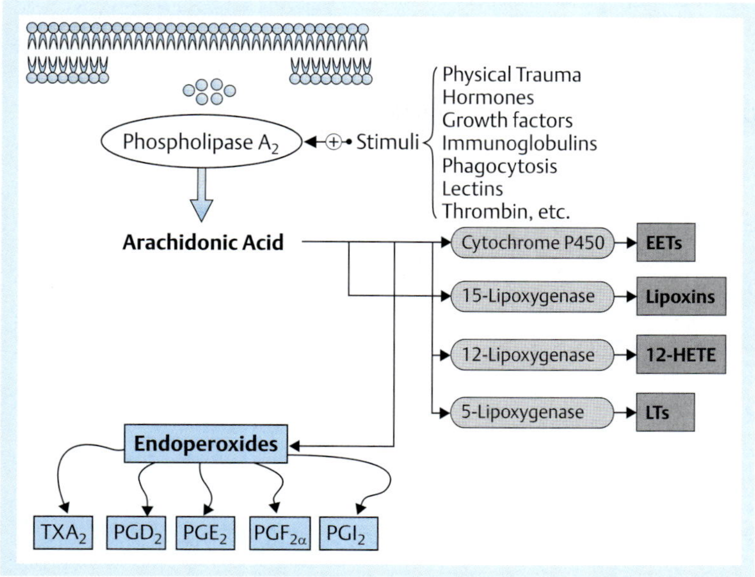

Fig. 2.**4** The prostanoid family. Epoxyeicosatrienic acids (EETs); 12-hydroxy-eicosatetraenoic acid (12-HETE); LTs: leukotrienes TXA_2: thromboxane A_2; PG: prostaglandins; PGI_2: prostacyclin.

an amino acid sequence of their complementary DNA showing only 60% homology, analogous enzymatic functions, and different tissue distribution, control mechanisms, sensitivity to inhibitors, and possibly physiologic functions [18, 19]. COX-1 contains 576 amino acids, COX-2 587 [19]. X-ray crystallography data have demonstrated that the overall topology of the enzymes is not affected by the minor variations in the amino acid residues observed between the two isoforms [20] and that the structures can be superimposed [20–22].

The tertiary structure of both isoforms (see Fig. 2.**6**), consisting of a long narrow channel with a hairpin bend at the end, includes three distinct domains: an N-terminal epidermal growth factor domain, a membrane-binding domain, and the C-terminal catalytic domain containing the cyclooxygenase and peroxidase active sites [20–22]. The cyclooxygenase active site is located at the end of a long, narrow hydrophobic channel [23].

COX-1 and COX-2 are membrane-associated enzymes and do not contain a transmembrane domain, but the membrane-binding domain comprises amphipatic helices that form a localized region of hydrophobicity that serves to anchor the lower portion of the enzyme in the membrane. The COX active site is located in an area of hydrophobicity near the amphipatic helices. Access to this site occurs via a channel buried in the lipid bilayer. Both substrates and inhibitors use this channel to reach the active site [20–22]. This structure allows arachidonic acid, which is released from membrane sites adjacent to the opening of the enzyme channel and is largely hydrophobic, to be drawn in and twisted around the hairpin bend. Two oxygens are then inserted and a free radical extracted, resulting in the five-carbon ring that characterizes prostanoids [22]. Nonsteroidal anti-inflammatory drugs (NSAIDs) inhibit cyclooxygenase activity by excluding access of arachidonic acid into the channel. X-ray crystallography has suggested that this blocking occurs by hydrogen bonding to the polar arginine at position 120. At position 523 there is an isoleucine molecule in COX-1 and a valine (smaller by a single methyl group) in COX-2. The smaller valine molecule in COX-2 leaves a gap in the wall of the channel, allowing access to a side-pocket, which is thought to be the binding site of many selective drugs. The bulkier isoleucine at 523 in COX-1 is large enough to block access to the side-pocket [24–27]. This difference at position 523 is compounded by the substitution of isoleucine 434 in COX-1 with a valine molecule in COX-2, within the second shell of amino acids surrounding the cyclooxygenase active site. This further increases the effective size of the active site channel by enhancing the mobility of side chains within the side pocket. The larger main channel combined with the extra nook increases the volume of the

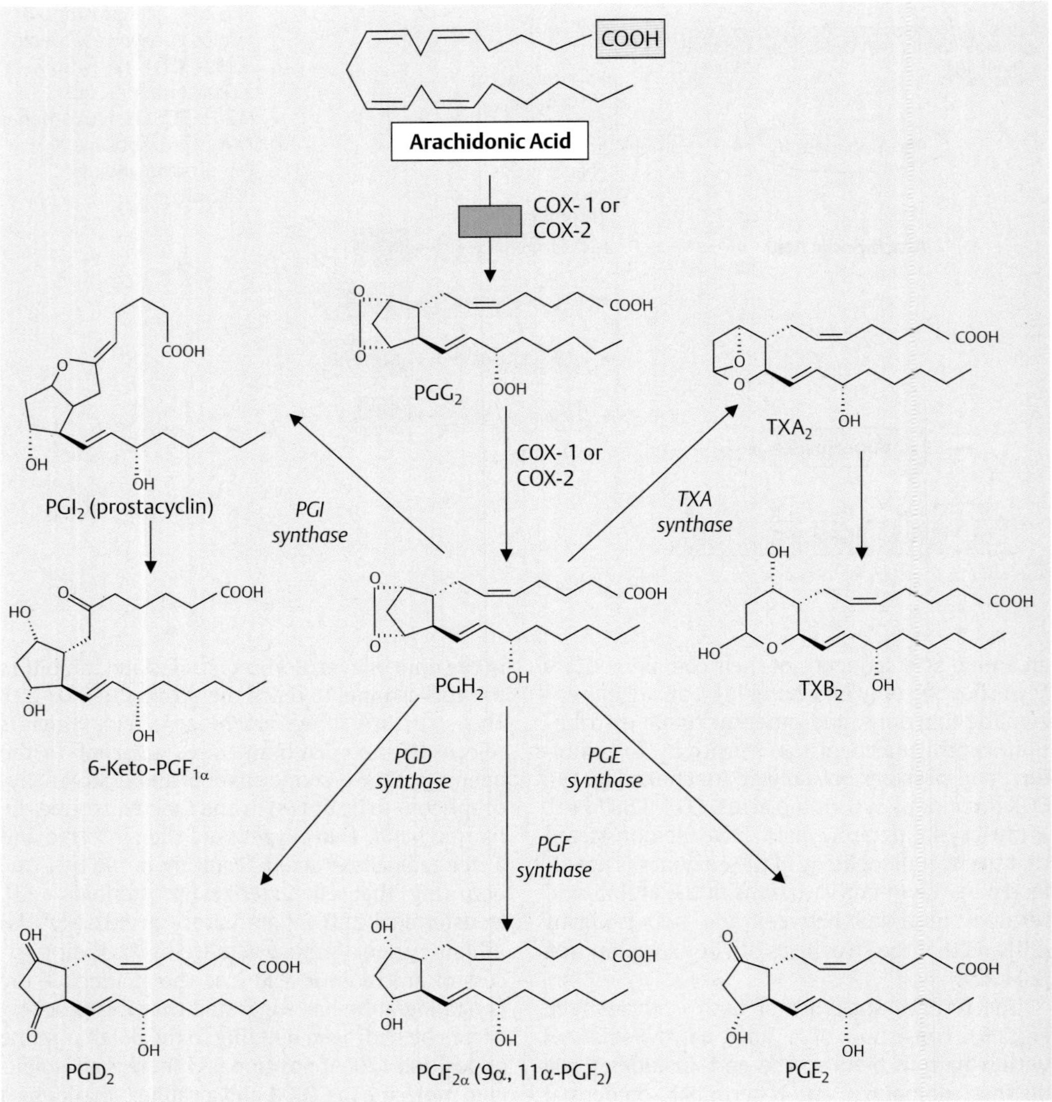

Fig. 2.**5** The cyclooxygenases pathway.

binding site of COX-2 NSAIDs by about 20% compared to the site in COX-1.

Localization of the COX isoforms

COX are membrane-associated enzymes, and in the cell membrane the two isoforms are equally distributed between the nuclear envelope and the endoplasmic reticulum membrane [28]. COX have also been observed in nonmembranous cytosolic lipid bodies, which accumulate in cells associated with inflammation, although the amounts of each COX isoform present in these organelles have not been determined [29].

The distribution of COX-1 and COX-2 in tissues under basal conditions has been well characterized by numerous tissue localization studies (northern blotting, immunohistochemical localization, in situ hybridization analyses). The COX-1 isoform can be found in nearly all tissues, including the gastrointestinal tract (GI), platelets, endothelial cells, and kidney [30], while COX-2 has

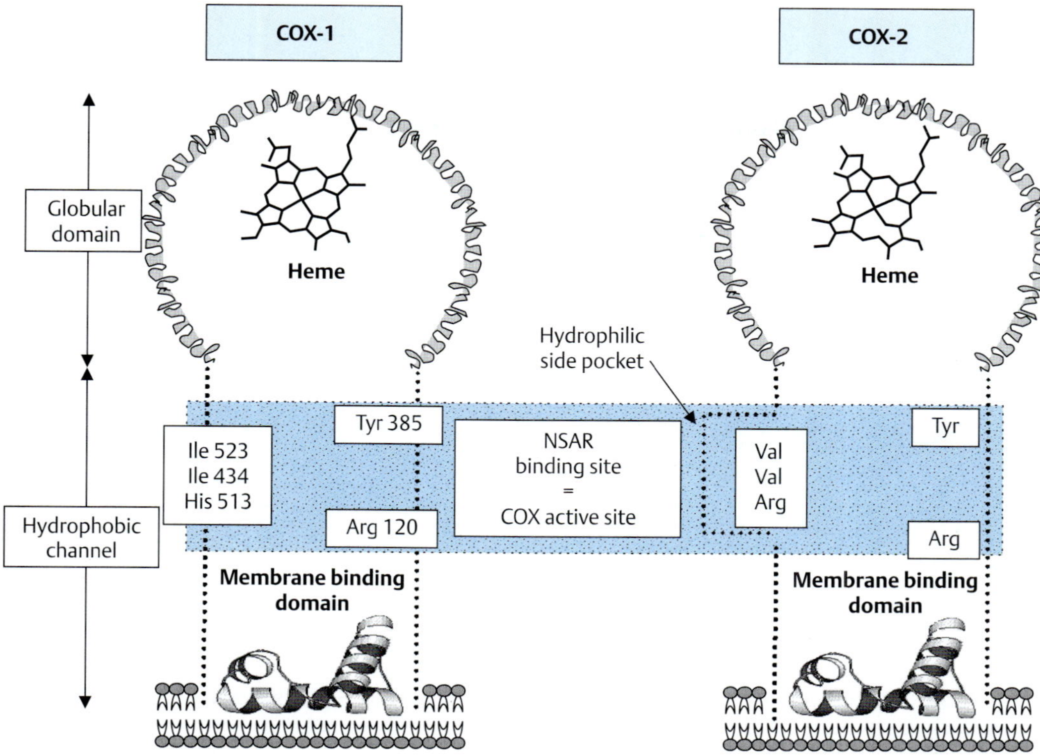

Fig. 2.**6** Schematic representation of the structure of cyclooxygenase-1 (COX-1) and cyclooxygenase-2 (COX-2).

been detected in the brain and kidneys and in small quantities in the lungs, liver, and stomach [31].

Considering the broad distribution of the COX-1 isoform, it can be considered a "constitutive" enzyme whose action mediates so-called "housekeeping" functions, such as regulation of the renal blood flow, gastric mucosal integrity, and platelet-dependent homeostasis. On the other hand, COX-2 is considered the "inducible" isoform that is normally absent from cells but is rapidly expressed in response to hormones, growth factors, pro-inflammatory cytokines, bacterial endotoxin, and tumor promoters [13, 18, 19].

Functions of the COX isoforms

As already stated, COX catalyzes two sequential reactions in spatially distinct but mechanistically coupled active sites. First, cyclooxygenases convert AA to PGG_2, removing a hydrogen atom, and thus generating an arachidonyl radical. Then peroxidase (a typical heme-dependent enzyme), reduces the hydroperoxide PGG_2 to PGH_2 [32].

Each COX isozyme catalyzes exactly the same reactions, producing the same products. The question arises as to why are there two COX isoforms and what roles they play.

Firstly, given that COX-1 is present in practically every tissue and is constitutively expressed, while COX-2 is highly inducible, COX-1 was thought to be primarily involved in cellular homeostasis, while COX-2 was thought to play a major role in inflammation, mitogenesis, and in various pathophysiologic processes. Furthermore, it was observed that the inhibition of COX-1 by compounds known as nonsteroidal anti-inflammatory drugs (NSAIDs) was related to the well-known side effects of these compounds, while the therapeutic actions were attributed to the inhibition of the COX-2 isozyme [13, 18, 19].

Further studies provide compelling evidence that ascribing exclusive "housekeeping" and inflammatory functions to COX-1 and COX-2, respectively, was an oversimplification.

The precise contributions of the two isoforms, in particular of the two COX genes, to various pathophysiologic processes was difficult to as-

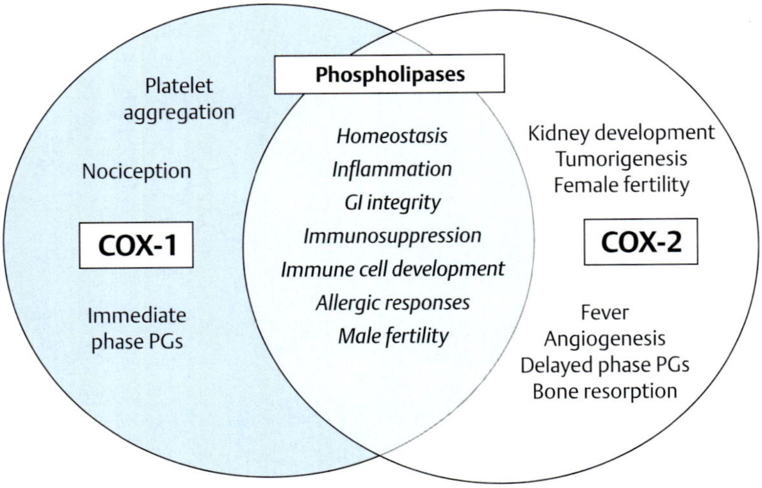

Fig. 2.**7** Functions of the COX isoforms. PGs: prostaglandins.

sess, but the use of mice in which one or the other of the COX genes were genetically "knocked out" has proved to be invaluable in deciphering the distinct biological roles of the two COX isozymes. These studies suggest that there are processes in which each isozyme is uniquely involved (e.g. platelet aggregation for COX-1, ovulation for COX-2), and others in which both isozymes act in consort (e.g. carcinogenesis, inflammation). There are also physiologic events that normally involve one COX but the other isoform can compensate if the first is lacking (e.g. parturition and remodeling of the ductus arteriosus).

Specific roles for the PGs generated by the two COX have been discovered in development, renal pathophysiology, reproduction, carcinogenesis, gastric ulceration, immune and inflammatory responses, regulation of body temperature, and nociception [13, 18, 19] (see Fig. 2.**7**).

Observations of mice with congenital COX deficiency have challenged the generally accepted concept that COX-1 is involved primarily in homeostatic/housekeeping functions, while the expression of COX-2 exclusively modulates inflammatory reactions. In fact, it could be argued that the basic effects of COX-1 and COX-2 deficiency on the mouse phenotype better supports the opposite conclusion, since ablation of the COX-2 gene causes more serious abnormalities than ablation of the COX-1 gene [33–35].

The physiologic processes of the two COX isozymes can be divided as follows [36] (see Table 2.**1**):

- Physiologic processes that depend primarily on COX-1,
- physiologic processes that depend primarily on COX-2,
- physiologic processes in which both COXs are involved and act in a coordinated manner.

COX-1-dependent physiologic processes

Platelet aggregation. Platelets synthesize thromboxane A_2 (TXA_2) from arachidonic acid (AA) generated from endogenous phospholipids stores. TXA_2 exits the cells and, via the platelet TXA_2 receptor (TP), initiates platelet shape modifications and subsequent platelet aggregation [37]. Acting through the same TP receptor, TXA_2 can also cause constriction of vascular smooth muscle. Platelets express only the COX-1 isoform, so that TXA_2 can be formed only by COX-1 [38]. In fact, COX-1-null mice fail to undergo AA-induced aggregation [39]; this also indicates that COX-2 cannot compensate for the absence of COX-1 in platelets. Low-dose aspirin used therapeutically as an antithrombogenic agent blocks COX-1-dependent platelet synthesis of proaggregatory TXA_2 without affecting endothelial cell synthesis of antiaggregatory prostacyclin (PGI_2) [40].

Parturition. The two COX isozymes play distinct physiologic roles in female reproduction. In COX-1-null female mice the litters were of normal size but difficulty with parturition occurred [39], whereas other aspects of the reproductive process were normal [41]. Other authors [42] also found that the onset of parturition was delayed in COX-1-null mice, and that administration of $PGF_{2\alpha}$ resulted in the onset of labor. This suggests that COX-1 is the isozyme responsible for the production of $PGF_{2\alpha}$. It was also observed in COX-1-null mice that under certain pathologic conditions COX-2 is able to compensate for the absence of COX-1 and produce the $PGF_{2\alpha}$ needed to initiate parturition [43].

COX-2-dependent physiologic processes

Ovulation and implantation. COX-2-null female mice are infertile [44]. Although follicular development is observed in COX-2-deficient mice, ovulation is greatly reduced and, of the eggs released, very few are fertilized [41]. Ovarian PGE_2 production is increased by pituitary gonadotropins in wild-type and COX-1-null mice but not in COX-2-null mice, indicating that COX-2 is responsible for this increased ovarian PGE_2 production. Because ovulation in COX-2-null mice can be restored by administration of PGE_2 [45]. This prostaglandin, formed via COX-2, is believed to be the product responsible for ovulation. In addition to affecting ovulation, COX-2 deficiency also impedes blastocyst implantation and decidualization. The prostanoid involved in this process is PGI_2, which is also synthesized by COX-2 [46].

Neonatal development. Even if it is believed that COX-1 acts in neonatal development, recent studies suggest that COX-2 plays a more important role in this process [47, 48]. COX-2-null mice develop severe renal pathology that is not mimicked by administration of NSAIDs to adult mice [44, 49]. Although this phenomenon represents a compensatory artifact of the COX-2 knockout, it has been recently shown that postnatal treatment with COX-2-selective NSAIDs caused a severe reduction in glomerular diameter in the neonatal mouse kidney. This is the same renal pathology seen in COX-2-null mice that cannot be produced by treating adult mice with COX-2-selective inhibitors [47]. COX-2 also has an essential role in the closure of the ductus arteriosus [48]. 35% of the COX-2-deficient mice died with a patent ductus within 48 hours of birth, while the other 65% survived to weaning, suggesting that COX-1 can play a compensatory role [36]. Indeed, a reduction in COX-1 gene dosage from wild type to heterozygosity further increases the incidence of patent ductus arteriosus and reduces the 48-hour survival of COX-2-null mice to about 20% [36].

Because the birthing processes involves a number of physiologic changes and stresses that can induce COX-2, and because COX-2-null mice have a reduced survival at all ages, it might be useful to investigate other neonatal tissue in which COX-2 induction promotes normal neonatal development.

Physiologic processes involving both, COX-1 and COX-2

Inflammation and wound healing. The relative contributions of the two isoforms to inflammatory response are incompletely resolved. Since the discovery of COX-2, this isozyme was considered responsible for production of the prostanoids involved in inflammation, but now there are studies which show that prostanoids formed by COX-1 are also implicated [39, 50, 51]. Furthermore, recent studies have demonstrated that COX-2 acts in both the initiation of the inflammatory response and the resolution phase of inflammation. In fact, in a rat model of carrageenan-induced pleurisy, there was a transient increase in COX-2 expression and in PGE_2 levels in the first phase of the inflammatory process; later, however, COX-2 was induced again to even higher levels and generated anti-inflammatory PGs, such as PGD_2 and 15-deoxy-$\Delta^{12,14}$-PGJ_2, but only low levels of the proinflammatory PGE_2 [51, 52]. In the same animal model it was found that late administration of a COX-2-selective inhibitor exacerbated the inflammatory response [52]. Moreover, in a carrageenan paw inflammation model the inflammation resolved within seven days in wild-type mice but it remained unmitigated over the same period in COX-2-null mice [51]. COX-2 therefore appears to have two roles in the inflammatory process, initially contributing to the onset of inflammation and later helping to resolve the process.

Gastric ulceration. For many years the gastrointestinal (GI) side effects of NSAIDs were thought to be related to the inhibition of the COX-1 isozyme, since constitutive expression of COX-2 in normal gastric mucosal tissue is low or absent [53]. In fact, it was surprising to discover that COX-1-null mice did not develop gastric ulcers spontaneously despite a 99% reduction in gastric PGE_2 levels [35, 39, 54, 55]. It was therefore pointed out that COX-2 may be involved in the so-called "adaptive cytoprotection" response in the GI mucosa [56] and may play a pivotal role in tissue-repair processes. It has been shown that

Table 2.1 Specific physiologic/pathologic functions of COX-1 and COX-2 [36]

Physiologic/pathologic process	COX-1	COX-2	PGs involved
Ovulation	NE	Essential	PGE_2
Implantation	NE	Essential	PGI_2
Parturition	Essential	Compensatory	$PGF_{2\alpha}$
Inflammation resolution	NE	Essential	PGD_2/15-deoxy-PGJ_2
Platelet aggregation	Essential	No role	TXA_2
Perinatal kidney development	NE	Essential	ND
Kidney function	Essential	Essential	PGE_2
Ductus arteriosus remodeling	Compensatory	Essential	TXA_2/PGH_2
T-cell development	Stage – specific	Stage-specific	PGE_2
Gastric ulceration	Inhibition	Inhibition	ND
Ulcer healing	NE	Essential	ND
Intestinal cancer	Essential	Essential	ND
Crypt stem cell survival	Essential	Compensatory	PGE_2

NE: not essential; ND: not determined

induction of gastric ulcers is associated with an increase in COX-2 mRNA production and mucosal prostaglandin synthesis. Treatment with a selective COX-2 inhibitor resulted in reduction in mucosal PG synthesis and significant inhibition of gastric ulcer healing in both mice [57] and rats [58]. Moreover, COX-2 is also involved in the production of angiogenic factors [59], a basic fibroblast growth factor that is localized in the fibroblast and capillary endothelium in granulation tissue and in the epithelium at ulcer margins [60]. Also, COX-2 induction has been demonstrated in *Helicobacter pylori* gastritis and in inflammatory bowel diseases and may be excessive as a result of subliminal bacterial infections of the gastric mucosa [61, 62]. Furthermore, the induction of gastric injury in rats by NSAIDs requires inhibition of both COX-1 and COX-2 [63]. Finally, the constitutive expression of COX-2 in healthy human and rabbit gastric mucosa has been described [64]. All this evidence directly challenges the concept that prostaglandins, important for maintaining GI mucosal integrity, are produced solely via COX-1.

Carcinogenesis. Most studies suggest that COX-2 rather than COX-1 is involved in colon carcinogenesis. However, it has been determined that deficiency of either COX-1 or COX-2 reduces polyp formation in *Min*$^{-/+}$ mice about equally (n. d. 80%) [65], raising the question of whether COX-1 and COX-2 contribute to tumorigenesis through shared or different mechanisms. It is possible that COX-1 functions in early stages of tumorigenesis by protecting initiated stem cells from damage-induced DNA death, while COX-2 contributes to tumor promotion after loss of heterozygosity of the APC gene [66, 67]. Other studies indicate that at the adenoma stage of tumor development COX-2 is present in the interstitial cells rather than the epithelial cells of the tumor. Thus, prostanoids formed via COX-2 exert a paracrine rather than an autocrine effect to promote tumor growth [65]. Selective COX-2 inhibitors have been shown to have clear antitumor efficacy in rodent models of adenomatous polyposis [68], to suppress growth, and to induce apoptosis in human esophageal adenocarcinoma cells [69]. Work with COX-null mice indicates that both isozymes contribute to the increased PGE_2 production seen in polyps. Overall, these results suggest that both COX isoforms play key roles in intestinal tumorigenesis and that COX-1 may also be an effective chemotherapeutic target for NSAIDs.

Immune response. PGs play a central role in mediating the immune response. In fact, they appear to modulate T-cell development and activation [70, 71]. Some authors [70, 71] have shown that COX-1 and COX-2 are both necessary for normal thymic T-cell maturation in the fetal mouse; both isozymes appear to play a distinct role in T-cell maturation and signal transduction via specific PG receptors. While both COX isoforms are expressed in the fetal thymus, their relative expression levels at each development stage vary significantly. For example, COX-1 is expressed predominantly in immature thymocytes, while COX-2 is highly expressed in the mature thymus. COX-2 expression in the developing thymus is localized to the medulla, while COX-1 expression appears to be restricted to the epithelial cells of the thymic cortex. Functionally, COX-1-mediated PGE_2 biosynthesis is thought to promote the transition of $CD4^-$ $CD8^-$ thymocytes to $CD4^+$ $CD8^+$ cells, acting via the EP_2 subtype receptor. COX-1 activity is essential for development of $CD4^+$ $CD8^+$ thymocyte population. On the other hand, COX-2-mediated PGE_2 biosynthesis and utilization of the EP_1 subtype receptor favor the selection and maturation of $CD4^+$ lymphocytes.

Interestingly, COX-1 inhibitors are more effective than COX-1 gene ablation in preventing the transition of lymphocytes from $CD4^-$ $CD8^-$ to $CD4^+$ $CD8^+$, suggesting that COX-2 may compensate for the lack of COX-1 in deficient mice, or that non-COX-related effects of these drugs can affect T-cell maturation. High COX-2 protein levels in the COX-$1^{-/-}$ thymus and a concordant increase in $CD4^+$ thymocytes is consistent with a compensatory mechanism.

Biochemical evidence for unique COX-1 and COX-2 biosynthetic pathways

For isozyme-specific effects to exist, COX-1 and COX-2 must be able to function independently at the biochemical level. This can be achieved if the isozymes are segregated into different cells. Often, however, the two isoforms are co-expressed in the same cells. Under the latter conditions, independent functioning of the COX isoforms appears to involve metabolic rather than physical separation of the enzymes. COX-1 and COX-2 are found mainly in the same organelles: at the luminal surfaces of the endoplasmic reticulum and in the nuclear envelope of cells [71], though it is likely that each isoform is restricted to a specific subdomain of these membranes.

When COX-1 and COX-2 are expressed in the same cells, supplying AA, either exogenously or via activation of cellular lipases, always leads to the functioning of COX-2. Only when COX-2 is absent does COX-1 appear to function independently. However, because COX-1 is a constitutive enzyme, while COX-2 is inducible, this is in fact the usual situation. COX-2 is usually present in cells only during early stages of cell differentiation or replication [72].

In cultured cells, the Km value of COX-1 for AA appears to be higher than that of COX-2 (~2 µM and 10 µM, respectively) [73, 74]. Moreover, the concentration of lipid peroxide required to activate the cyclooxygenase activity of COX-1 is about ten times greater than that necessary for COX-2 in the presence of low AA concentrations [36]. Thus, a combination of low endogenous peroxide concentrations within the lumen of the endoplasmic reticulum, where COX-1 and COX-2 are predominately localized in intact cells [71], and AA concentrations below 2 µM [75, 76] would favor the activities of COX-2 over those of COX-1. Thus, regardless of the mechanism, it appears that the activities of COX-1 and COX-2 are controlled differentially by regulating the amount of lipid peroxide and AA available to the enzymes. Another way in which COX-1 and COX-2 biosynthetic pathways may be dissociated metabolically is via preferential coupling of the two isozymes to various downstream synthases, e.g. TXA_2 synthase, PGI_2 synthase, and/or microsomal PGE (mPGE) synthase [72, 77, 78]. In fact, COX-2 appears to be coupled metabolically to PGI_2 formation in the uterus in association with decidualization and implantation, and there also appears to be an mPGE synthase that is coordinately induced with COX-2 and appears to function preferentially with COX-2 rather than COX-1 [79, 80]. Also, the coupling of the two COX isozymes with different PLA_2 forms could play a role in this regulation. $cPLA_2$ is involved in mobilizing AA for COX-1, but prostaglandin formation during the late phase involving COX-2 depends on both $cPLA_2$ and one or more $sPLA_2$ [78, 81, 82–84].

2.4 Products of the cyclooxygenases: prostaglandins and thromboxanes

Structure, receptors, downstream enzymes, metabolism and catabolism, and functions

Structure. Prostaglandins and thromboxanes fal into several main classes designated by letters and differentiated by substitutions on the cyclopentane ring. Prostaglandins of series E and D are hydroxyketones, while F_α prostaglandins are 1,3-diols. PGI_2 has a two-ringed structure; in addition to the cyclopentane ring, a second ring is formed by an oxygen bridge between carbon atoms 6 and 9. TXs contains a 6-member oxane ring rather than the cyclopentane ring of the PGs.

These main classes are further subdivided by use of a subscript number, which refers to the number of double bonds in the side chains. This is indicated by subscript 1, 2, or 3 and reflects the fatty acid precursor in most instances. Dihomo-γ-linolenic acid is the precursor of the one series, arachidonic acid of the two series, and eicosapentenoic acid of the three series. Prostaglandins and thromboxanes derived from arachidonate carry the subscript 2 and constitute the major prostanoids in mammals.

Receptors. Prostanoid receptors are cell-specific and are named according to the natural prostanoid for which they have the greatest affinity. They are divided into five principal classes: DP receptor for PGD_2, EP receptor for PGE_2, FP receptor for PGF_2, IP receptor for PGI_2, and TP receptor for thromboxane A_2. Of these receptors, EP has been divided into four subtypes: EP_1, EP_2, EP_3, EP_4, and four splice variants of EP_3 have been described which appear to have different signal transduction mechanisms [85, 86].

All prostanoid receptors so far identified are coupled to effector mechanisms through a G_s protein [87, 88], and two second-messenger systems are associated with their action: 1) adenylate cyclase stimulation/inhibition with consequent increase/reduction of intracellular cyclic AMP (cAMP) levels; and 2) phospholipase C activation with subsequent increased formation of diacylglycerols and inositol-1,4,5-triphosphate, responsible for increases in cytosolic Ca^{2+} concentrations.

Several prostanoids, including 15-deoxy-$\Delta^{12,14}$-prostaglandin J_2 and a variety of nonsteroidal anti-inflammatory drugs (NSAIDs) bind to peroxisome proliferator-activated receptors (PPARs) [89, 90], members of the nuclear hormone receptor superfamily. Three subclasses of PPAR have been described: PPARα, PPARβ and PPARγ. The metabolic oxidation pathways activated by PPARs ligands metabolize lipid mediators such as PGs and leukotrienes, so that PPARs ligands have been considered as possible anti-inflammatory agents acting through the enhanced breakdown of proinflammatory prostanoids. Thus, affinities for these receptors are significantly weaker than for membrane receptors, and their binding is associated with suppression of the elaboration of inflammatory products [91 – 93]. This is a further demonstration that some prostanoids exhibit not only inflammatory but also anti-inflammatory activities.

Downstream enzymes. The synthase enzymes that convert the endoperoxide products of COX into the primary prostanoids PGE_2, PGD_2, $PGF_{2\alpha}$ PGI_2, and TXA_2 have been characterized relatively recently.

PGE synthase. An inducible PGE synthase [94] recently identified is a 15 – 16-kDa glutathione-dependent, membrane-associated protein that is upregulated by interleukin-1β (IL-1β) and downregulated by phenobarbitone. PGE synthase and COX-2 are likely to be co-induced by cytokines such as IL-1β, so that PGE_2 biosynthesis may depend on the activity of both of these enzymes [95, 96]. However, two separate glutathione-dependent PGE synthases with different tissue and subcellular distributions have been reported:

1. A cytosolic PGE synthase found mainly in the brain that might predominantly convert PGH_2 derived from COX-1 to PGE_2;
2. A microsomal PGE synthase induced during the inflammatory response that may be functionally linked with COX-2 in preference to COX-1 [97].

PGF synthase. PGF synthase is a 36.8-kDa cytosolic enzyme isolated from bovine and human lungs and from bovine liver. It not only catalyzes the reduction of PGH_2 to $PGF_{2\alpha}$ but also reduces PGD_2 to 9α, 11β-PGF_2 [98, 99]. This enzyme belongs to the aldo-keto reductase family, and the lung and liver types differ in terms of substrate concentration, kinetics, regulation by metals, sensitivity to chloride ions, and immune-precipitation profile [100].

PGD synthase. There are two types of PGD synthase that catalyze the isomerization of PGH_2 to PGD_2; the hematopoietic type and the lipocalin type [101]. The former is a glutathione-dependent enzyme that was purified from rat spleen and is expressed in several tissues and cell types, such as mast cells, megakaryoblastic cell lines, histiocytes, etc. In humans, it is expressed strongly in the placenta, less so in the lungs, and weakly in the brain. The latter are members of a superfamily of lipophilic ligand-carrier proteins binding, including retinoids and thyroid hormones. The two types differ in terms of catalytic properties, amino acid sequence, tertiary structure, origin, gene structure, chromosomal and cellular localization, and tissue distribution [101].

TXA synthase. TXA synthase is a 58.8-kDa membrane-bound protein attached to the endoplasmic reticulum [102] and containing 533 amino acids. It catalyzes the conversion of PGH_2 to TXA_2, which degrades chemically within 30 s to thromboxane TXB (TXB_2), the stable but inactive hydrolysis product [102, 103]. The highest concentrations of TXA synthase are found in platelets, followed by blood monocytes. TXA synthase activity is also found in many other tissues, such as the lungs, kidneys, and spleen as well as in macrophages and fibroblasts. TXA synthase is a hemoprotein, and its primary structure shows a 34–36% similarity to the amino acid sequences of cytochrome P450 (CYP450).

PGI synthase. PGI synthase catalyzes the final conversion of PGH_2 to PGI_2, a bicyclic prostanoid with a short chemical half-life which undergoes hydrolysis to the inactive substance 6-keto-$PGF_{1\alpha}$. PGI synthase is a membrane-bound hemoprotein that is predominantly expressed in vascular endothelium and smooth muscle cells [104] and in many human tissues, particularly in the ovary, heart, skeletal muscles, lungs, and prostate gland. Its amino acid sequence is about 32% homologous with the sequences of the P450 enzymes but shares only 16% common identity with the structure of thromboxane synthase.

Metabolism and catabolism. The first products of the catalytic action of the COX isozymes are the prostaglandins PGG_2 and PGH_2. As mentioned earlier, PGH_2 is chemically unstable and can be transformed enzymatically into a variety of compounds, including PGI_2, TXA_2, PGE_2, $PGF_{2\alpha}$, and PGD_2 (see Fig. 2.**8**). Although most tissues are able to synthesize the PGH_2 intermediates from free arachidonate, their providence varies in each tissue and depends on the complement of enzymes present and their relative abundance.

TXA_2 is produced mainly by activated platelets, while the PGI_2 form found in vascular endothelial cells (which counteracts the biological effects of TXA_2) and other PGs are produced by a variety of cell types.

In platelets PGH_2 is metabolized by thromboxane synthase into thromboxane A_2 (TXA_2), which then breaks down nonenzymatically into the stable but inactive TXB_2. In vascular endothelium cells the metabolic transformation of PGH_2 leads mainly to the synthesis of prostacyclin (PGI_2) via prostacyclin synthetase. PGI_2, in turn, is nonenzymatically hydrolyzed to the inactive 6-keto $PGF_{1\alpha}$. In macrophages PGE_2 is mainly formed, while mast cells express chiefly PGD_2 (see Fig. 2.**8**). Tissues such as the spleen and lungs are able to synthesize the entire range of AA cascade products.

Prostanoids must be removed quickly from the tissues, and, in fact, efficient mechanisms exist for their catabolism and inactivation. Generally, there are two enzymatic types of catabolic reactions: a relatively rapid initial enzymatic stage, catalyzed by widely distributed prostaglandin-specific enzymes, whereby the PGs lose most of their biological activity, and a second, relatively slow enzymatic stage, in which the metabolites are oxidized by enzymes that are probably identical to those responsible for β and ω oxidation of most fatty acids.

The initial stage is the oxidation of 15-OH dehydrogenase (PGDH). The 15-keto compound is then reduced to the 13,14-dihydro derivative, a reaction catalyzed by prostaglandin Δ^{13}-reductase. Subsequent steps consist of β and ω oxidation of the side chains of PGs, giving rise to a polar dicarboxylic acid, which is excreted in the urine as the major metabolite of both PGE_1 and PGE_2 (see Fig. 2.**8**).

Unlike PGE_2, PGD_2 is initially reduced to the F-ring prostaglandin 9α, 11β-PGF_2 and PGI_2 is hydrolyzed to 6-keto-$PGF_{1\alpha}$. These two compounds then undergo metabolism similar to that of other prostanoids (see Fig. 2.**8**).

TXA_2 is rapidly hydrolyzed to TXB_2 and then oxidated; many metabolites have been identified in the urine but the most abundant are 2,3-dinor-TXB_2 and 11-dehydro-TXB_2 (see Fig. 2.**8**). These reactions take place mainly in the liver.

Functions

Prostanoids may have diverse physiologic and pathologic functions, and in fact play a major role in the following (see Table 2.**2**):

- Platelet aggregation and homeostasis
- Reproduction and parturition
- Vascular and pulmonary smooth muscle
- Kidneys
- Inflammation, pain, fever, immune system and cancer
- Gastrointestinal tract
- Brain

Platelet aggregation and homeostasis. Stimulation of platelet aggregation causes activation of membrane phospholipases with the consequent liberation of AA and its transformation into thromboxane A_2, which amplify platelet aggregation and produces vasoconstriction. Conversely, PGI_2 produced in the cells of the vessel wall potently inhibits platelet aggregation and

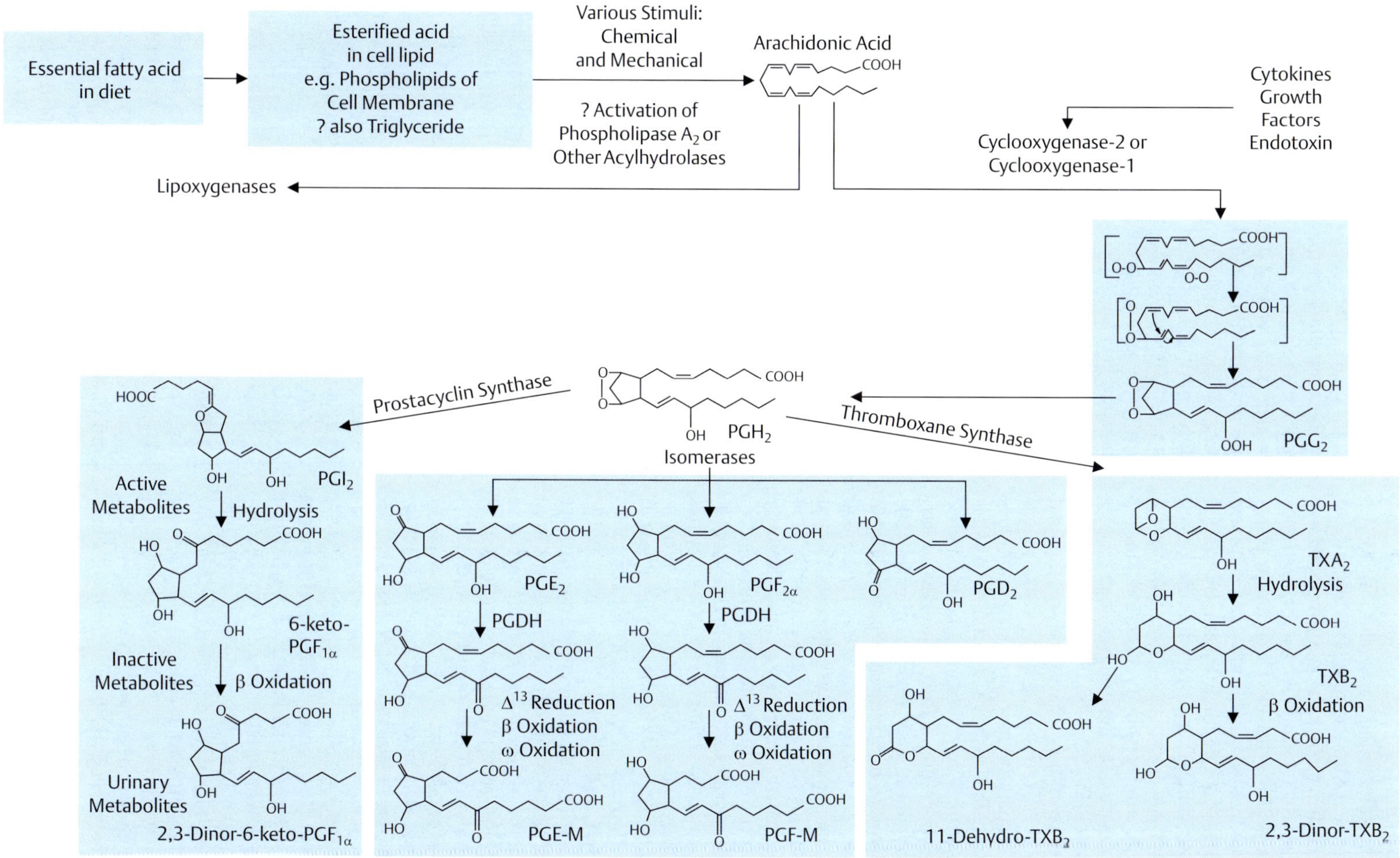

Fig. 2.**8** Products of the catalytic action of the COX isozymes.

contributes to the nonthrombogenic properties of the vascular endothelium. It also induces vasodilation via relaxation of the smooth muscle of the blood vessel walls. PGI_2 and TXA_2 therefore represent biologically opposite poles of a mechanism for regulating platelet-vessel wall interactions and the formation of homeostatic plugs and intra-arterial thrombi [105].

Reproduction and parturition. Several PGs, including PGE_2 and $PGF_{2\alpha}$, certainly play an important role (though this has not yet been fully clarified) in the physiology of reproduction. The observation of elevated concentrations of prostaglandins in human sperm, associated with the fact that they are absorbed by the vaginal walls, has led to the belief that prostaglandins deposited in the vagina during coitus may facilitate conception by acting upon the cervix, body of the uterus, fallopian tubes, and transport of the seminal fluid. In fact, some correlation has been observed between low concentrations of prostaglandins in sperm and male infertility. Before and during menstruation there is an increase in prostaglandin synthesis, which may induce painful contractions of the myometrium and sensitize the afferent pain fibers, producing dysmenorrhea. Nonsteroidal anti-inflammatory drugs have been shown to be highly efficacious in this pathologic condition. During pregnancy the production of prostaglandins gradually increases, and the concentration of these substances is very high in blood and amniotic fluid during labor. It is not clear, however, if they are responsible for the onset of labor or if they contribute to the maintenance of uterine contractions initiated by oxytocin. It is known that COX inhibitors prolong pregnancy, delay the onset and prolong the duration of labor. Prostaglandins and prostaglandin analogs are also useful in preparing the cervix for delivery and as abortifacients. Additional evidence for a role of PGs in reproduction and parturition is provided by the fact that targeted disruption of the genes encoding both COX enzymes, the EP_2 receptor, and the FP receptor in mice results in various defects in parturition and reproduction [106].

Vascular and pulmonary smooth muscle. Locally generated PGE_2 and PGI_2 modulate vascular tone. They may play an important physiologic role in the maintenance of sufficient blood flow to vital organs, in maintaining adequate placental blood flow during pregnancy, and in maintaining patency of the arterial duct in the fetus.

The airway contracts in response to $PGF_{2\alpha}$ TXA_2, and PGD_2, whereas PGE_2 and PGI_2 are weak bronchodilators. PGD_2 and $PGF_{2\alpha}$ potentially constrict the airways in asthmatic patients and potentiate the constrictor response to other spasmogens [107, 108]. Raised levels of bronchoconstrictor PGs in the lungs may therefore contribute to allergic bronchospasm during asthmatic attacks. $PGF_{2\alpha}$ and TXA_2 constrict pulmonary blood vessels, but in some species PGE_2 causes dilation. PGI_2 is a potent vasodilator in the pulmonary circulation in humans and other species and may be important in regulating vascular pulmonary tone in chronic hypoxia.

Mediators of inflammation, such as histamine, 5-hydroxy-tryptamine, and bradykinin, release PGs from lung tissue. Proinflammatory cytokines, such as tumor necrosis factor-α (TNF-α) and IL-1β, are present in the inflamed airways of asthmatic patients [109] and induce COX-2 expression in pulmonary epithelial and endothelial cells, smooth muscle of airways, and alveolar macrophages [110]. PGE_2 is the main product of COX-2 induced in the lung epithelial cells [111, 112], and *in vitro* studies in animals suggest that it may protect against bronchoconstriction induced by endothelin, bradykinin, and tachykinins [113–117]. Thus, endogenous PGE_2 may be bronchoprotective in asthma and may act as an anti-inflammatory factor [118]. Aspirin-induced asthma may be triggered by increased release of leukotrienes from inflammatory cells caused by removal of the inhibitory influence of PGE_2, the major product of COX-2 in the airways [119–121].

Kidneys. The renal cortex produces mainly PGE_2 and PGI_2 with very small amounts of TXA_2 [122], while the renal medulla produces mostly PGE_2. PGE_2 and PGI_2 are vasodilators and increase renal blood flow. Their formation is increased by factors that reduce renal blood flow (angiotensin, catecholamine). Prostaglandins are also natriuretic, inhibiting tubular reabsorption of sodium and, in the thick ascending limb of Henle they reduce chloride transport. In the renal cortex PGE_2 and PGI_2 are important stimulators of renin release, and the PGI_2 formed by COX-2 in mesangial cells may directly stimulate renin secretion. Bartter's syndrome (a rare disease characterized by low-to-normal blood pressure, decreased sensitivity to angiotensin, hyperreninemia, hyperaldosteronism, and excessive loss of potassium) has been attributed to increased biosynthesis of prostaglandins; in fact, many symptoms dimin-

Table 2.**2** Physiologic and pathologic functions of prostanoids

PGs	Function	Organ/System
PGE_2	Vasodilatation	Arterioles, precapillary sphincters, postcapillary venules, gastric mucosa vessels
	Vasoconstriction	Some vessels
	Decreasing blood pressure	Arteries
	Increase of blood flow	Heart, kidneys, splanchnic viscera
	Increase of cardiac output	Heart
	Relaxation of smooth muscle	Bronchial, tracheal, nonpregnant uterus, and at high concentrations in pregnant uterus; circular muscles of the GIT
	Contraction	Pregnant uterus at low concentrations; main longitudinal muscles of the GIT
	Diarrhea and abdominal cramps	GIT
	Reduction of the volume of secretion, acidity and content of pepsin	Stomach
	Increase of mucus secretion	Stomach
	Increase of diuresis, natriuresis and kaliuresis	Kidneys
	Secretion of renin via a direct effect on granular juxtaglomerular cells	Renal cortex
	Hyperalgesia	Nerves
	Increase of circulation of ACTH, growth hormone, prolactin, gonadotropin	Endocrine
PGD_2	Vasodilatation	Vascular region at low concentrations
	Vasoconstriction	Vascular region at high concentrations; pulmonary circulation
	Contraction	Bronchial and tracheal smooth muscles
	Secretion of renin via a direct effect on granular juxtaglomerular cells	Renal cortex
	Somnogen, nociceptive modulation	Nervous system
$PGF_{2\alpha}$	Vasoconstriction	Pulmonary arteries and veins, arteries of the endometrium
	Increase of cardiac contractility Modulation of cardiac rhythm Increase of cardiac output	Heart
	Contraction of smooth muscle	Bronchi and trachea, pregnant and nonpregnant uterus, GIT
PGI_2	Vasodilatation Hypotension Bronchodilation	Vessels, bronchial smooth muscle
	Increase of cardiac output	Heart
	Inhibition of platelet aggregation	Platelets
	Relaxation	Myometrium of pregnant uterus
	Contraction	GIT

continuation next page

Table 2.**2** Physiologic and pathologic functions of prostanoids *(continuation)*

PGs	Function	Organ/System
PGI_2	Reduction of the volume of secretion, acidity and content of pepsin	Stomach
	Increase of mucus secretion	Stomach
	Increase of diuresis, natriuresis and kaliuresis	Kidneys
	Secretion of renin via a direct effect on granular juxtaglomerular cells	Renal cortex
	Hyperalgesia	Afferent nerves
TXA	Vasoconstriction	Vessels, lungs, kidneys
	Aggregation	Platelets
	Contraction	Myometrium of nonpregnant uterus, GIT
	Glomerular filtration decrease	Kidneys

GIT: gastrointestinal tract

ish following prolonged administration of cyclooxygenase inhibitors.

Inflammation, pain, fever, immune system and cancer. Prostaglandin production is stimulated by a whole series of insults: mechanical, thermal, chemical, bacterial, and others and greatly contributes to the signs and symptoms of inflammation. Though PGs do not appear to have direct effects on vascular permeability, PGE_2 and PGI_2 markedly enhance edema formation and leukocyte infiltration by promoting blood flow in the inflamed region. They also can sensitize nociceptors on sensory nerve terminals to painful stimulation, and, they also potentiate the algesiogenic effect of other autacoids, particularly bradykinin and histamine [123]. In addition, fever is caused by the release of PGE_2 by inflammatory mediators in the blood vessels of the hypothalamus [124]. PGE_2 synthesis close to the organum vasculosum lamina terminalis (OVLT) region of the hypothalamus is stimulated by the cytokine IL-1, whose formation is stimulated by the lipopolysaccharide (LPS) from infecting organisms. It is therefore likely that PGI_2 and PGE_2 contribute to the development of inflammatory erythema, pain [125], and fever [124].

PGD_2, produced almost exclusively by mast cells, is an allergic and inflammatory mediator.

No known prostanoids are produced by lymphocytes, although both COX isozymes have been detected in these cells [126].

In macrophages the release of PGE_2 may act as a negative feedback control mechanism, reducing further activation and producing inhibition of the immune function. PGE_2 inhibits interleukin-2 (IL-2) and interferon-γ (IFN-γ) production from T lymphocytes as well IL-1 and tumor necrosis factor-α (TNF-α) release from macrophages; it also induces the differentiation and maturation of immature thymocytes and B-lymphocytes [127–130]. PGE_2 produced by tumor cells accounts for depression of the immune system associated with cancer. In rheumatoid arthritis inhibition of PGs formation by NSAIDs leads to the removal of their immunosuppressant effect. Another consequence of removing suppression of the immune process by PGs may be the enhancement of cartilage breakdown [131, 132].

It should be pointed out that PGsE inhibit the participation of lymphocytes in delayed hypersensitivity reactions and the liberation of hydrolases and lysosomal enzymes by neutrophils. In fact, though, PGsE play an important role in the termination of inflammation by inhibiting the activation of macrophages, and the production and liberation of inflammatory cytokines. Prostaglandins also inhibit the immune response, the survival of skin grafts/transplants being prolonged by the administration of prostaglandins.

Certain spontaneous human tumors (medullary carcinoma of the thyroid, renal-cell adenocarcinoma, carcinoma of the breast), are accompanied by increased concentrations of local or circulating PGs, bone metastasis, and hypercalcemia. Some studies have implicated the effects of prostaglandins on either the hematogenous metastasis of tumors or on tumor angiogenesis. In experimental animals various PGs induce proliferation of colon cancer cells, and COX inhibitors reduce colon tumor formation. In large epidemiological studies regular use of aspirin was associated with a decreased incidence of colon cancer in humans, and COX inhibitors significantly decreased polyp formation in patients with familial colon polyposis syndromes.

Gastrointestinal (GI) tract. The cytoprotective action of prostaglandins is complex, and depends on a combination of several mechanisms. PGE_2 and PGI_2 reduce the secretion of gastric acid by the parietal cells of the stomach and increase gastric mucosal blood flow by direct vasodilator action. PGE_2 stimulates the release of viscous mucus [133] that could play a defensive role against mucosal injury [134]. Mucus release, other than providing a physical barrier, may act to create an unstirred layer of secreted bicarbonate [135] and therefore help neutralize hydrogen ions diffusing back from the lumen into the mucosa.

Brain. COX-1 is found in neurons throughout the brain, but it is most abundant in the forebrain [136, 137] where PGs may be involved in complex integrative functions, such as control of the autonomic nervous system and sensory processing. Low levels of COX-2 protein and COX-2 mRNA have been detected in forebrain neurons without previous stimulation by proinflammatory stimuli [136, 137, 138]. These "basal" levels of COX-2 are particularly high in neonates and are probably induced by nervous activity. PGE_2 is synthesized in the human brain, as is PGD_2, which has a rather limited distribution. Large amounts of PGD_2 are found in the brains of mammals [139, 140] and in mast cells but practically nowhere else. PGE_2 and PGD_2 have opposing actions in sleep and temperature regulation. While PGD_2 injected into the preoptic area of the rat brain induces normal sleep [141], PGE_2 infused into the region of the posterior hypothalamus causes wakefulness [142]. Similarly, administration of PGD_2 lowers body temperature [143], while PGE_2 has a pyretic action [144].

NSAIDs: nonsteroidal anti-inflammatory drugs

Anti-inflammatory, analgesic, and antipyretic drugs are a heterogeneous group of often chemically unrelated compounds which are categorized according to their certain therapeutic actions and side effects. They are frequently called *nonsteroidal anti-inflammatory drugs*, or *NSAIDs*, and, because the prototype is aspirin, they are also often referred as aspirin-like drugs. The main mechanism of action of aspirin and NSAIDs is the inhibition of the COX isozymes responsible for the formation of prostaglandins and thromboxanes. The drugs generally do not inhibit the formation of other prostanoids, such as leukotrienes, which also contribute to inflammation, nor do they affect the synthesis of numerous other inflammatory mediators.

Aspirin acts by covalently modifying both COX isozymes and therefore results in irreversible inhibition of COX activity. As a consequence, the duration of the effects of aspirin is related to the turnover rate of cyclooxygenases in various target tissues.

Unlike aspirin, most NSAIDs act as reversible competitive inhibitors to block COX activity. In this case the duration of their action is primarily related to the pharmacokinetic clearance of the drugs from the body.

Because aspirin and related drugs are organic acids, they accumulate at sites of inflammation, which is an attractive pharmacokinetic property for drugs intended as anti-inflammatory agents.

As explained earlier, COX-1 is thought to be the constitutive enzyme, responsible for the production of PGs with specific physiologic "housekeeping" functions, while COX-2 is the inducible isoform, produced in inflamed tissues. Thus, NSAIDs are thought to exert their therapeutic effect by inhibiting COX-2 and to produce adverse side effects, mainly gastrointestinal and renal effects, by inhibiting COX-1 activity.

Therapeutic effects

NSAIDs, including selective COX-2 inhibitors, have analgesic, antipyretic, and anti-inflammatory properties. One exception is acetaminophen, which is antipyretic and analgesic but is largely devoid of anti-inflammatory activity. This can be explained by the fact that the substance effectively inhibits COX in the brain but not at sites of inflammation in peripheral tissues.

NSAIDs, like analgesics, are usually only effective against pain of low-to-moderate intensity. Though their maximal analgesic effects are much weaker, NSAIDs lack the unwanted side effects of opioids on the central nervous system.

NSAIDs do not alter the perception of sensory modalities other than pain. Chronic postoperative pain and pain arising from inflammation are particularly well controlled by NSAIDs, while pain arising from the hollow viscera is usually not relieved.

NSAIDs as antipyretics lower the body temperature in febrile conditions. The fact that selective COX-2 inhibitors are effective antipyretic agents indicates that COX-2 is the COX isoform predominantly involved in thermoregulation.

These drugs are used as anti-inflammatory agents in the treatment of musculoskeletal disorders, such as rheumatoid arthritis, osteoarthritis, and ankylosing spondylitis. Generally speaking, NSAIDs provide only symptomatic relief of pain and inflammation associated with the disease but do not arrest the progression of the pathologic injury to tissue.

Other uses of NSAIDs depend upon the drugs' capacity to block prostaglandin and thromboxane biosynthesis. The release of $PGF_{2\alpha}$ from the endometrium during menstruation produces contraction of uterine smooth muscle and constriction of endometrial arterioles, which may be the causes of severe cramps and other symptoms of primary dysmenorrhea; treatment of this condition with NSAIDs has met with considerable success [145].

Prostaglandin D_2 released from mast cells in large amounts has been found to be the major mediator of severe episodes of vasodilatation and hypotension in patients with systemic mastocytosis. Treatment with antihistamines alone is usually ineffective, while the addition of an NSAID usually leads to effective prevention of these episodes [146, 147]. PGE_2 has also been implicated in humoral hypercalcemia associated with some neoplasms, and treatment with NSAIDs can effectively suppress serum calcium levels in some cancer patients [148].

Prostaglandins have been implicated in the maintenance of patency of the ductus arteriosus, and indomethacin and related agents have been used in neonates to close the ductus when it remained patent.

Aspirin at low doses has the capacity to inhibit platelet cyclooxygenase and therefore TXA_2 for the life of the platelet (8 to 11 days). This is the mechanism of action by which it exerts its antiaggregating effect in the prophylactic treatment of thromboembolic disorders. An important area where the use of NSAIDs is emerging is in the prevention of colon cancer. There is a compelling body of evidence suggesting that the effect of NSAIDs on colon cancer is mediated by inhibition of COX-2, which is markedly upregulated in colon tumors [149].

Side effects

NSAIDs also share several unwanted side effects, the induction of gastrointestinal injury, such as gastric and/or intestinal erosion and/or ulceration with consequent blood loss and anemia, being the must common. This side effect may be due to local irritancy on the gastrointestinal mucosa but especially to systemic inhibition of the biosynthesis of gastric PGs (PGI_2 and PGE_2), which act as cytoprotective agents on the gastric mucosa [150].

NSAIDs have unwanted side effects on renal function which are especially evident in some pathologic conditions, such as congestive heart failure, hepatic cirrhosis, chronic renal disease, etc. As already seen, prostaglandins exert important functions in the kidneys. Inhibition of their production by NSAIDs decreases renal blood flow and glomerular filtration rate and provokes water and sodium retention, causing peripheral edema. The response to diuretic therapy may also be reduced, and usually moderate increases in blood pressure are sometimes observed. Hyperkalemia is another electrolyte disturbance that can occur as a result of inhibition of PG synthesis. The effects of NSAIDs on electrolyte and water homeostasis appear to be dose-dependent [151, 152]. Acute renal failure is a rare but potentially serious complication of NSAID therapy and is mediated hemodynamically as a result of decreased renal perfusion following inhibition of PGI_2 synthesis.

Nephritic syndromes and papillary necrosis are very rare renal adverse effects. Acute interstitial nephritis may develop at any time during NSAID therapy and is usually combined with minimal change glomerulonephritis. The mechanism by which NSAIDs may induce nephritis, is greater availability of AA for metabolic pathways producing leukotrienes [153, 154], which increase vascular permeability in the glomerular and peritubular capillaries, leading to proteinuria and interstitial nephritis. Renal papillary necrosis is the least common but potentially most severe NSAID-related renal adverse event, as it results in permanent renal parenchymal damage.

The gastrointestinal and renal side effects of NSAIDs appear to be related to the drugs' inhibition of COX-1. However, it has recently been shown that these unwanted side effects are due to inhibition of both isoforms. In fact, COX-2 is not only an inducible enzyme but it is also constitutively present in several organs, where it participates with COX-1 in maintaining homeostasis, while COX-1 may be induced and contribute to the inflammatory response.

Platelet function is impaired because NSAIDs prevent platelets from synthesizing TXA_2, a potent aggregating agent. This accounts for the ability of these drugs to prolong bleeding time. Aspirin in particular is an effective inhibitor of platelet function, because the irreversible effect on COX activity requires new platelet production for restoration of enzyme activity. This "side effect" has been used in the prophylactic treatment of thromboembolic disorders. It also has been seen that acute administration of a selective COX-2 inhibitor suppresses the production of PGI_2 by about 80% without inhibiting TXA_2 formation and platelet aggregation [155]. This finding suggests that COX-2 is a major source of PGI_2 production *in vivo*. Since an important action of PGI_2 is thought to be the suppression of platelet activation, alteration of the TXA_2/PGI_2 ratio which accompanies selective inhibition of COX-2 is theoretically prothrombotic. However, even if it remains to be determined whether or not this is clinically relevant, it may be prudent to consider these findings when choosing an NSAID for the treatment of patients who are particularly prone to thrombotic events.

Certain individuals display intolerance to aspirin and most NSAIDs; this is manifested by symptoms that range from vasomotor rhinitis, angioneurotic edema, generalized urticaria, and bronchial asthma to laryngeal edema, bronchoconstriction, flushing, hypotension, and shock. The mechanism underlying this hypersensitivity reaction to NSAIDs is not known, but a common factor appears to be the ability of these drugs to inhibit COX activity. This has prompted the hypothesis that the reactions reflect the diversion of AA metabolism toward the formation of increased amounts of leukotrienes and other products of the LOX pathway, which are a thousand times more potent than histamine and induce bronchoconstriction, vasodilatation, vasopermeability, mucus secretion, and leukocyte chemotaxis.

Another potential side effect seen with the use of NSAIDs is an elevation of mean blood pressure (BP). The mechanisms responsible for increased BP related to treatment with NSAIDs include effects on both blood volume and peripheral resistance. As discussed above, inhibition of renal PG synthesis can lead to water and sodium retention, thus increasing plasma volume, as well as inhibition of prostacyclin synthesis, which is a potent vasodilator and under certain conditions may increase peripheral resistance. Another hypothesis to explain the effects of NSAIDs on BP postulates increased synthesis of endothelin-1, which has the capacity to induce salt and water retention and may have a systemic effect on BP by increasing peripheral vascular resistance.

The relative contribution of COX-1 and COX-2 isoforms in the production of PGs that are important for BP regulation are not known, but data from clinical trials of coxibs indicate that these compounds have similar effects on blood pressure as traditional NSAIDs.

Other side effects of NSAIDs resulting from the inhibition of endogenous prostaglandin synthesis include prolongation of gestation or spontaneous labor and premature closure of the patent ductus.

COX-2 inhibitors

Given the widespread use of NSAIDs, gastrointestinal and renal toxicity is the most prevalent drug-associated health risk. This has stimulated a search for selective COX-2 inhibitors, which promise to have the same anti-inflammatory, antipyretic, and analgesic activities as classical NSAIDs but are not expected to cause the same side effects, especially at the GI level.

Some NSAIDs with a limited degree of COX-2 selectivity were already available or under development before the notion of an inducible COX was introduced. These compounds have more favorable safety profiles than classical NSAIDs, and it has been demonstrated that they preferentially inhibit COX-2, although they are not devoid of COX-1 inhibitory activity [156]. Examples of such COX-2 preferential inhibitors include nimesulide, meloxicam, and salicylic acid. Nimesulide is between 5 and 16 times more selective for COX-2 than for COX-1 [26,157]; meloxicam has been estimated to be between 3 and 77 times more selective for COX-2 [158,159]. Two other NSAIDs, etodolac and nabumetone, may be COX-2 selective, but the available evidence is less well developed [160,161,162]. Of the first-generation NSAIDs, only diclofenac approaches equipotency in terms of its effects on COX-1 and COX-2 [163,164]; all other existing NSAIDs tend to be predominantly COX-1 selective [24].

NSAIDs that have emerged from drug-development programs based on an understanding of the differences between COX-1 and COX-2 have a higher selectivity for COX-2, which means that they inhibit COX-2 but have a limited or insignificant effect on COX-1 over the whole range of doses used and at the concentrations achieved in clinical treatment [164]. Drugs classified as highly selective COX-2 inhibitors include compounds such as celecoxib and rofecoxib.

Based on human recombinant-enzyme assays, celecoxib is quoted as being 375 times more selective for COX-2 than for COX-1, although it may be less selective in other assays [165, 166]. Clinical studies have shown that it is as effective in reducing arthritic pain and inflammation as ibuprofen and diclofenac in osteoarthritis and rheumatoid arthritis. The use of this drug was associated with a significantly lower incidence of GI adverse effects compared with standard NSAIDs in nonaspirin users [167].

Some authors suggest that celecoxib exhibits relative rather than absolute biochemical selectivity for COX-2 at doses tolerated in humans [168].

Another selective COX-2 inhibitor is rofecoxib, which is more than 800 times more selective for COX-2 [169, 170]. In human whole-blood assay samples from individuals receiving single doses of rofecoxib the estimated IC_{50} for COX-2 was 0.77 µM, while the IC_{50} for COX-1 could not be calculated because inhibition was not seen with single doses up to 1000 mg (i.e. 40 to 80 times the recommended therapeutic dose). Other studies using human whole blood assays have shown that rofecoxib selectively inhibits COX-2 in a dose-dependent manner, with little inhibitory effect on COX-1 [171]. Rofecoxib at a daily dose of 50 mg was found to be of similar efficacy to naproxen and ibuprofen and superior to placebo in postoperative dental pain ($p < 0.01$) [172]. In patients with osteoarthritis rofecoxib was found to be significantly more effective than placebo and similar in clinical efficacy to diclofenac, ibuprofen, and nabumetone but with a lower incidence of gastrointestinal adverse events [173].

The incidence of myocardial infarction was lower among patients taking naproxen than among those taking rofecoxib (0.1 vs 0.4%); however, the overall mortality rate and the rate of death from cardiovascular events were similar in the two groups [174]. Preliminary studies with rofecoxib indicate that COX-2-selective inhibitors have effects on renal functions similar to those of traditional nonselective NSAIDs, in particular on sodium homeostasis [175]. Renal effects are more evident in patients with diminished renal function or in situations, such as a sodium-restricted diet, where renal dependence on PG production is enhanced [176, 177]. On the basis of the experimental and clinical data available so far, the equation COX-2 selectivity = more effective and safer NSAIDs is widely claimed, especially at the GI level. However, recent data have cast some doubts on the effects of long-term treatment with these highly selective inhibitors. As already stated, studies with COX knockout mice suggest that PGs formed by both COX isoforms are involved in the inflammatory response, while those generated by COX-2 contribute substantially to regulation of many physiologic functions, such as, gastric ulcer healing, renal function, reproductive physiology, and resolution of inflammation.

Also, the need for more comprehensive clinical investigations of selective COX-2 inhibitors to ascertain their potential side effects is reinforced by postmarketing surveillance reports for rofecoxib. A newsletter from the Medicine Control Agency and the Committee on Safety of Medicines reported that an estimated 557,100 prescriptions for rofecoxib have been dispensed in the UK up to the end of May 2000, and a total of 1120 reports of suspected adverse reactions to the drug were received by the agencies. The majority (84%) were GI reactions, while there were 177 reports of suspected cardiovascular reactions. Adverse reactions common to classical NSAIDs, e.g. angioedema, bronchospasm, exacerbation of asthma, renal failure, and hepatic dysfunction, were also reported [13].

Therapeutic and side effects

Gastrointestinal tract. COX-2 is present in the stomach [178], and COX-2 induction has been demonstrated in *Helicobacter pylori*-related gastritis and in inflammatory bowel disease, and COX-2 may be overexpressed as a result of subliminal bacterial infections of the gastric mucosa [179, 180]. Thus, specific inhibitors of COX-2 may become harmful in the presence of gastrointestinal inflammation. In fact, COX-2 may be involved in the so-called "adaptive cytoprotection" response in gastrointestinal mucosa [181].

A number of recent studies have evaluated the effects of COX-2-selective drugs in animal models of pre-existing gastrointestinal inflammation. In a rat model of colitis the majority of prostaglandins produced by the colonic mucosa are derived from COX-2 [182]. Daily treatment with a selective COX-2 inhibitor at doses that do not inhibit

COX-1 resulted in significant inhibition of mucosal prostaglandin synthesis and a marked increase in the severity of colonic damage [182]. When treatment was continued for a week, colonic ulceration was exacerbated resulting in perforation of the bowel and death in 100% of the rats [182].

COX-2 is rapidly induced in GI ulcerative processes, where it generates large amounts of prostaglandins that contribute to the healing process. Administration of selective COX-2 inhibitors results in significant inhibition of gastric ulcer healing in both, mice [183] and rats [184]. It is noteworthy that the ulcer healing inhibition was observed with doses previously shown to produce selective inhibition of COX-2 [185]. Moreover, induction of gastric injury in rats by NSAIDs requires inhibition of both COX-1 and COX-2 [186]. There is also a report which demonstrated the constitutive expression of COX-2 in healthy human and rabbit gastric mucosa [187]. All these data challenge the concept that the PGs important for the maintenance of GI mucosal integrity are not produced only via COX-1.

Resolution of inflammation. Recent data indicate that even if prostanoids are among the principal initiators of the inflammatory reaction, they might also function as anti-inflammatory mediators with a role in terminating the process. In a variety of nonimmune and immune inflammatory models it was noted that there was an early rise in PGE_2 levels, which correlated with the onset of inflammation, and a fall during resolution, followed by a rise in levels of $PGF_{2\alpha}$ as inflammation decreased. The latter was able to inhibit increased vascular permeability induced by other mediators, such as histamine and serotonin. It was therefore suggested that a change in PG synthesis pathways occurs during the resolution of inflammation, consequently altering the PG profile [188, 189–191]. Moreover, in the rat model of carrageenan-induced pleurisy two peaks of COX-2 activity were observed, at 2 and 48 hours. The second peak of expression, which was 350% greater than that at 2 hours, was associated with minimal PGE_2 synthesis and coincided with resolution of the inflammatory reaction. In contrast, at 48 hours a peak was observed in the synthesis of anti-inflammatory prostanoids such as 15-deoxy-Δ^{12-14}-PGJ_2. Indomethacin and a selective COX-2 inhibitor reduced inflammation at 2 hours but significantly exacerbated inflammation at 48 hours. Thus, COX-2 may be proinflammatory during the early phases of the inflammatory process, but may contribute to resolution of the inflammation in a later phase by generating anti-inflammatory prostanoids [192, 193].

It has also been reported that inhibitors with selectivity for COX-1 were more effective than COX-2-selective drugs [194], and with some highly selective COX-2 inhibitors a significant anti-inflammatory effect was observed after administration of doses that also inhibit COX-1. This suggests that, despite not being induced, COX-1 appears to contribute substantially to prostaglandin synthesis in inflammation [195].

Renal function. Maintenance of renal function in patients with congestive heart failure, liver cirrhosis, or renal insufficiency is dependent on PGs with a vasodilator action. These patients are therefore at risk for renal ischemia when prostaglandin is reduced by NSAIDs [196]. Synthesis of PGE_2 and prostacyclin is mainly by COX-1, but COX-2 is also involved [197]. Moreover, upregulation of COX-2 expression has been observed in the macula densa after salt deprivation and appears to be important in the control of renin release [197]. It is not unlikely that COX-2 inhibitors share the effects of nonselective NSAIDs on renal function. Yet available data obtained in experimental models suggest an even more important role for COX-2 than for COX-1, especially in kidney development.

Reproductive function. COX-2-null female mice are infertile [44]. Although follicular development is observed in COX-2- deficient mice, ovulation is greatly reduced and, of the eggs released, very few are fertilized [198]. Ovarian PGE_2 production is increased by pituitary gonadotropins in wild-type and COX-1-null mice but not in COX-2-null mice, indicating that COX-2 is responsible for such increased ovarian PGE_2 production. Because ovulation in COX-2-null mice can be restored by administration of PGE_2, this prostaglandin formed via COX-2 is believed to be the product responsible for ovulation. In addition to affecting ovulation, COX-2 deficiency also impedes blastocyst implantation and decidualization. The prostanoid involved in this process is PGI_2, which is also synthesized by COX-2.

Although it is believed that COX-1 figures in neonatal development, recent studies suggest that COX-2 plays a more important role in this process [47, 48]. COX-2-null mice develop a severe renal pathology that is not mimicked by the administration of NSAIDs to adult mice [44, 49], suggesting that this phenomenon is a compensatory artifact of the COX-2 knockout. However, it has been recently shown that postnatal treatment with COX-2-selective NSAIDs causes a severe reduction in glomerular diameter in the neonatal mouse kidney – same renal pathology seen in COX-2-null mice that could not be caused by treating adult mice with COX-2-selective inhibitors [47]. COX-2 also has an essential role in the closure of the ductus arteriosus [48]. Uterine COX-2 is induced at the end of pregnancy and is important for the onset of labour [199].

These data suggest that specific inhibitors of COX-2 are likely to share the effects of nonselective NSAIDs on ovulation and parturition.

Cardiovascular function. The effects of COX-2 inhibitors on the incidence of vascular diseases also require scrutiny, particularly considering that COX-2 is a major source of prostacyclin biosynthesis in humans [168]. COX-2-specific inhibitors could increase the thrombotic risk because they block the production of PGI_2 (a potent anti-aggregating agent), but, since they do not inhibit COX-1, do not block the formation of TXA_2 released from platelets, thus favoring a prothrombotic state. Further studies will be necessary to evaluate whether these compounds are contraindicated in patients at risk of stroke or heart attacks.

Finally, COX-2 specificity limits the therapeutic applications of COX-2 inhibitors. These agents will not replace the cardiovascular protective effects of nonselective NSAIDs which are mediated through COX-1 inhibition.

2.5 Lipoxygenases

Recent evidence indicates that a number of mediators other than COX-activated products are involved in producing and maintaining inflammation. In fact, an important role in inflammation is played by products of the lipoxygenases pathways of arachidonic acid metabolism (see Fig. 2.**9**), in particular by leukotrienes (LT_S) (see Fig. 2.**10**).

Lipoxygenases (LOX) are a family of cytosolic enzymes that catalyze the oxygenation of polyunsaturated fatty acids (PUFA). They contain two *cis* double bonds separated by a methylene group [200]. Three mammalian LOX have been purified cloned, expressed, and classified according to the position at which they oxidize AA, i.e. 5-lipoxygenase (5-LOX), 12-lipoxygenase (12-LOX), and 15-lipoxygenase (15-LOX). Of these enzymes the most biologically important is arachidonate-5-lipoxygenase [200]. All three enzymes are able to oxygenate AA and other PUFA with the requisite 5-carbon unit. The initial oxygenation of AA by these LOX leads to the formation of hydroperoxyeicosatetraenoic acids (HPETEs), such as 5-*S*-HPETE, 12-*S*-HPETE, and 15-*S*-HPETE [200]. Like the endoperoxides PGG and PGH, HPETEs are highly reactive, short-lived intermediates which are transformed to monohydroxyeicosatetraenoic acids (HETEs) by peroxidases, such as glutathione peroxidase [200].

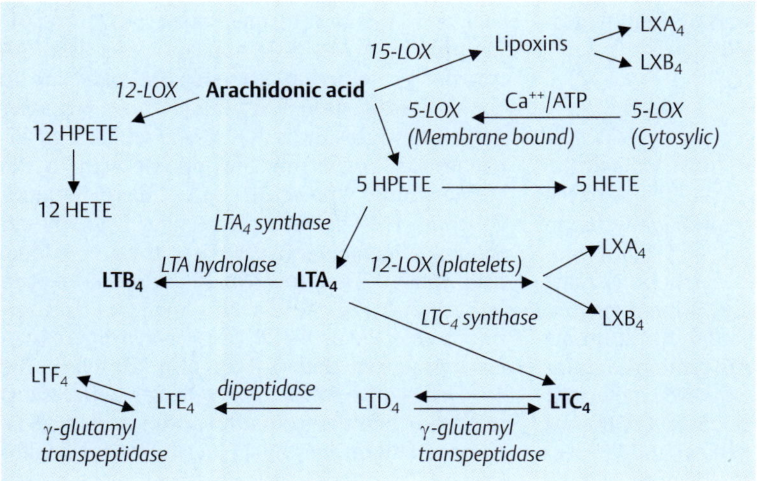

Fig. 2.**9** Lipoxygenases pathways.

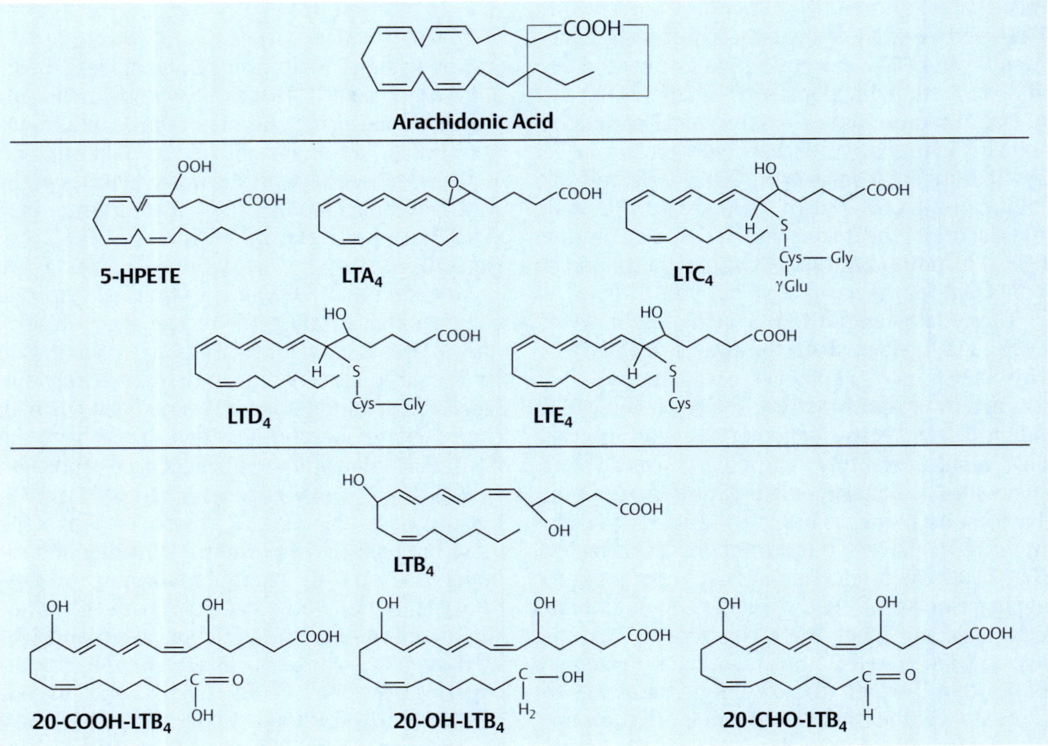

Fig. 2.**10** Lipoxygenase products and their structure.

Lipoxygenases: category, localization and functions

As mentioned above, three mammalian lipoxygenases exist. Each is found in various cell types and catalyzes the oxygenation of polyunsaturated fatty acids to the corresponding lipid hydroperoxides (see Figs. 2.**9** and 2.**10**).

5-lipoxygenase (5-LOX)

5-lipoxygenase is perhaps the most biologically important of the lipoxygenases, as it leads to the synthesis of leukotrienes. It is principally found in cells of myeloid origin, such as polymorphonuclear leukocytes, macrophages, eosinophils, mast cells, monocytes, basophils, and B-lymphocytes, that are involved in inflammatory and immune reactions. 5-LOX is a monomeric protein containing a nonheme iron, with an estimated molecular weight of between 72 and 80 kD. 5-LOX cDNA has been cloned from various species, and the sequences show more than 90% identity. Human 5-LOX contains 674 amino acids, is hydrophobic, and lacks signal sequences. 5-LOX activity is dependent on Ca^{2+} and ATP, a characteristic that differentiates this enzyme from other LOX.

When cells are activated and intracellular Ca^{++} increases, 5-LOX, which is normally present in the cytoplasm, translocates to the nuclear envelope and links to transmembrane 5-LOX activating protein (FLAP). FLAP appears to act as an AA transfer protein that presents the substrate to the 5-lipoxygenase [200, 201]. Thus, 5-lipoxygenase catalyzes the initial step in leukotriene biosynthesis, converting arachidonic acid to the stereospecific molecule, (5*S*)-*trans*-5,6-oxido-7,9-*trans*-11,14-*cis*-eicosatetraenoic acid, by removing a molecular hydrogen at the arachidonic acid carbon-7, and inserting a molecular oxygen at carbon-5 [202–205]. This molecule is commonly referred as 5-HPETE, or 5-hydroperoxyeicosatetraenoic acid. 5-LOX also catalyzes the stereospecific removal of a hydrogen with radical migration and the formation of the unstable 5,6-epoxide leukotriene A_4 (LTA_4), the parent leukotriene [202–205]. LTA_4 conversion to the potent chemoattractant leukotriene B_4 (LTB_4) is catalyzed by the enzyme leukotriene A_4 hydrolase, while the conjugation of LTA_4 with reduced glutathione to form LTC_4 is catalyzed by the enzyme LTC_4 synthase [202–205]. γ-glutamyltranspeptidase catalyzes the conversion of LTC_4 to LTD_4. Leukotriene D_4 is biologically more potent than leukotriene C_4, being converted to LTE_4 by the action of LTD_4 dipeptidase. LTC_4, LTD_4, and LTE_4 are also called peptidoleukotrienes or cysteinyl-leukotrienes [202–205].

12-lipoxygenase (12-LOX)

This enzyme has been found in human platelets, human erythroleukemia cells, and endothelial cells of the human umbilical vein. This arachidonate-12-lipoxygenase catalyzes the transformation of arachidonic acid to 12-HPETE, which may also be molecularly rearranged and transformed to form epoxyhydroxyeicosatrienoic acids, called hepoxylins [200].

15-lipoxygenase (15-LOX)

Arachidonate-15-lipoxygenase, has been found in human eosinophils, alveolar macrophages, monocytes, and epithelial cells. It is controlled and regulated primarily by IL-4 and IL-13 [206, 210], two cytokines that are implicated as negative regulators of the inflammatory response or anti-inflammatory cytokines. 15-LOX catalyzes the biosynthesis of 15-HPETE, which is subsequently transformed by neutrophils into trihydroxylated metabolites called lipoxins that play an important role as anti-inflammatory molecules.

2.6 Leukotrienes: structure, receptors and functions

Structure and receptors

As already stated, activation of PLA_2 induces mobilization of essential fatty acids from the membrane lipid pool, especially arachidonic acid, for the synthesis of lipid mediators at the site of cellular damage. Arachidonic acid is metabolized by two major pathways to proinflammatory mediators: the COX-pathway and the 5-LOX pathway. As discussed above, 5-LOX, which is present in the cytoplasm of the cell, after binding to the transmembrane protein FLAP catalyzes a two-step reaction (see Figs. 2.**9** and 2.**10**), oxygenation of arachidonate at the fifth carbon to form 5-HPETE, which, in turn, is partially transformed to the unstable LTA_4, and 5-HETE.

As with prostaglandins, a subscript is used to indicate the number of double bonds in the fatty acid. Arachidonic acid is the precursor of the four series of leukotrienes, and 5,8,11,14,17-eicosapentaenoic acid the precursor of the five series. Also, like PGs, leukotrienes have profound effects on a wide variety of tissues, and these effects are mediated via specific membrane receptors. Three different *leukotriene receptors* have been identified, the LTB_4 receptor (BLT), and two cysteinyl-LT receptors (CysLT1 and CysLT2) [211]. Only the BLT receptor has been cloned [212]; it is a seven-transmembrane-spanning receptor, which especially mediates chemotaxis [212, 214]. The CysLT1 and CysLT2 receptors have been characterized pharmacologically but not structurally [214]. Most of the actions of the cysteinyl-LT receptors are mediated by the CysLT1 receptor [214], including the contraction of human airway smooth muscle, chemotaxis, and increased vascular permeability.

The signal transduction of leukotriene receptors appear to be linked to the turnover of inositol phosphates via activation of phospholipase C. Regulation of the activity of phospholipase C appears to be coupled to the receptor via a guanine-nucleotide-binding protein [211, 215, 216].

Leukotriene A_4 (LTA_4) is the unstable intermediate for the synthesis of the other LTs, and it is produced only in cells of myeloid origin in which 5-LOX is expressed. However, it can also be released from activated leukocytes [217, 218] and taken up by adjacent cells devoid of 5-LOX activity but expressing the other enzymes (LTA_4-hydrolase and LTC_4-synthase) necessary for the synthesis of LTs. This process is called *transcellular biosynthesis* [219–221] and allows the amplification of LT production in inflamed tissues. LTA_4-hydrolase and LTC_4-synthase are enzymes much more widely distributed than 5-LOX. LTA_4-hydrolase is a cytosolic enzyme responsible for the transformation of LTA_4 to 5,12-dihydroxyeicosatetraenoic acid, known as LTB_4. LTC_4-synthase is the only enzyme that synthesizes peptido-LTC_4. This enzyme has a high selectivity for its substrate, a microsomal localization, and its activity appears to be modulated by a number of cytokines, including IL-3, IL-5, granulocyte-macrophage-colony stimulating factor (GM-CSF), and transforming growth factor-β (TGF-β) [222–224]. Transformation to LTC_4 involves the conju-

Table 2.**3** Specific biological effects of leukotrienes

Leukotriene	Function	Organ/cell
LTB_4	Chemotaxis	Polymorphonuclear leucocytes, eosinophils and monocytes
	Aggregation	Neutrophils, eosinophils
	Recruitment, migration, adhesion	Polymorphonuclear leukocytes
	Degranulation with superoxide generation	Polymorphonuclear leukocytes
	Increase cytokine production and release	Polymorphonuclear leukocytes
	Increase cytotoxicity and cytokine production (IL-5, IL-6, IL-8)	T lymphocytes Macrophages (?)
	Inhibition of proliferation and release of lymphokines	T lymphocytes
	Increase of proliferation, activation and immunoglobulin production	B lymphocytes
	Permeability increase	Microvasculature
	Hyperalgesia	Afferent nerves
LTC_4, LTD_4, LTE_4	Contraction	Smooth muscle peripheral airways, large arteries or veins, coronary arteries, distal segments of the pulmonary artery, gastric mucosa vasculature, gastrointestinal smooth muscle
	Mucus secretion and mucosal edema	Bronchi
	Increase permeability	Microvasculature
	Recruitment of inflammatory cells	Lymphocytes, eosinophils
	Stimulation of secretion of glycoproteins	Lungs
	Airway remodeling in chronic allergic inflammation	Lungs

gation of LTA_4 with reduced glutathione. LTD_4 is then produced by the removal of the glutamic acid from LTC_4, and LTE_4 results from the subsequent cleavage of glycine by the enzyme LTD_4-dipeptidase. Reincorporation of glutamic acid yields a glutamylcysteinyl derivative called LTF_4 (see Figs. 2.**9** and 2.**10**). LTC_4, LTD_4, and LTE_4 are also called peptidoleukotrienes or cysteinyl-leukotrienes and collectively make up the slow-reacting substances of anaphylaxis (SRS-A).

Functions

Leukotrienes are potent mediators of inflammation. Their specific biological effects are summarized in Table 2.**3**.

Leukotrienes in disease states

Leukotrienes are potent mediators of inflammation and are involved in the pathogenesis of a wide variety of human inflammatory diseases, such as rheumatoid arthritis, osteoarthritis, gout, psoriasis, inflammatory bowel disease, asthma, and hypersensitivity reactions. Each of these enzymes contributes to the inflammatory response through a variety of biological effects which will be described next.

Leukotriene B_4

LTB_4 causes neutrophil, lymphocyte, monocyte, and eosinophil chemotaxis, neutrophil and eosinophil aggregation, neutrophil degranulation, lysosomal enzyme release, neutrophil-endothelial cell adhesion, modulation of pain induced by inflammatory reactions, and modulation of certain immune responses. In part, these responses may be mediated through the generation of cell proinflammatory cytokines, such as interleukin-1β (IL-1β) and tumor necrosis factor-α (TNF-α). It has been explained that activation of nuclear factor kB (NF-kB) – the transcription factor responsible for the expression of pro-inflammatory cytokines, such as TNF-α, and of adhesion molecules – requires reactive oxygen intermediates produced by the 5-lipoxygenase-cascade [222]. Thus, stimulation of the nuclear factor kB signaling cascade by LTB_4 has been documented and is probably responsible for mediating the LTB_4-dependent transcriptional effects on COX-2 and IL-1. Proinflammatory cytokines, particularly TNF-α and IL-1β, play a cardinal role in the pathophysiology of arthritic diseases [223, 224]. Leukotrienes are powerful stimulators of proinflammatory cytokine synthesis. In fact, they have been implicated as important mediators of chronic inflammation and joint destruction in experimental models of rheumatoid arthritis [225] and osteoarthritis (OA) [223]. Moreover, LTB_4 was detected in significant quantities in the synovial fluid and joint tissue of untreated control animals with OA and rheumatoid arthritis [223, 226, 227].

It has recently been shown [228] that the coronary vasoconstriction observed in arthritic rats is associated with increased activity of the 5-lipoxygenase system in the heart and with a consequently increased local production of leukotrienes (LTB_4 and LTC_4). LTB_4 has been recovered from skin-lesions of patients with active psoriasis.

LTB_4 is the most obvious candidate for the inflammatory lesions created by neutrophils observed in colonic and small-bowel mucosa in ulcerative colitis and Crohn's disease. Actually, human colonic epithelial cells are capable of synthesizing LTs, and LTB_4 levels are elevated in colonic mucosa biopsies removed from patients with these two disorders [229, 230].

Although the physiologic role of leukotrienes in the kidneys is not well established, increased levels have been observed in many renal diseases. LTs are synthesized in the kidney by infiltrating leukocytes or macrophages, possibly with the secondary intervention of renal resident cells. Leukotrienes have a number of biologic actions that may be specifically relevant to the pathogenesis of renal disease [231]. LTB_4 stimulates chemotaxis, promotes leukocyte adhesion to endothelial cells, and modulates interleukin-1 production. In animal models of immune-mediated glomerulonephritis LTB_4 has been associated with neutrophil infiltration and degranulation in the glomeruli. Increased renal levels of LTB_4 were observed in rat models of membranous nephropathy [232] and in nephrotoxic serum nephritis [233]. Infusion of LTB_4 results in a reduction of renal blood flow and glomerular filtration rate [227]. Thus, increased synthesis of this lipid mediator within the kidneys during disease states may promote glomerular inflammation and injury.

Cysteinyl-leukotrienes (LTC_4, LTD_4 and LTE_4)

The cysteinyl-leukotrienes have powerful spasmogenic actions, especially in smooth muscle of airways and in the vasculature and are released during asthmatic attacks, in inflammation, in rheumatoid arthritis, and in hypersensitivity reactions. LTC_4 has been recovered in the nasal lavage fluids of patients with allergic rhinitis during both the early and the late phases of inflammation following allergen challenge [234, 235]. When administered by aerosol, these mediators are at least 100 times more potent than histamine as bronchoconstrictors in man [236].

LTC_4 and LTD_4 have been recovered from skin-lesions of patients with active psoriasis and from intestinal mucosa of patients with ulcerative colitis or Crohn's disease [229, 230].

Leukotrienes are also responsible for gastric injury. In fact, at the GI level they cause increased vascular permeability, resulting in mucosal microvascular injury, gastric vasoconstriction, breakdown of the mucosal barrier, accumulation and activation of leukocytes, and increased production of proinflammatory cytokines. Vasoconstriction in the gastric mucosa causes a significant reduction of blood flow and accounts for the ulcerogenic effects of cysteinyl-leukotrienes [227]. Some experimental data support the postulate that, besides causing a reduction in the synthesis of vasodilatory and gastroprotective prostaglandins, COX inhibition by NSAIDs diverts arachidonate acid to the 5-lypoxygenase pathway, thus increasing the formation of LTB_4 and cysteinyl-leukotrienes [237, 238]. This causes vasoconstriction of the gastric mucosa and increases the formation of reactive oxygen radicals from the peroxidative cleavage of HPETEs [239] with additional mucosal injury. Indeed, NSAID-induced gastric and intestinal mucosal lesions are prevented by the concurrent administration of 5-lipoxygenase inhibitors [237, 238].

Table 2.**4** Involvement of the various leukotrienes in some pathologic states

Leukotriene	Species	Pathologic state	Localization
LTB_4	Human	Rheumatoid arthritis Gout	Synovial fluid
		Psoriasis	Skin lesion
		Ulcerative colitis, Crohn's disease	Colonic mucosa
		Mesangial proliferative nephritis	Kidneys
	Animals	Glomerular immune injury	Kidneys
	Rat	Membranous nephropathy	Kidneys
		Nephrotic serum nephritis	Kidneys
Cysteinyl-leukotrienes (LTC_4, LTD_4 and LTE_4)	Human	Allergic rhinitis	Nasal lavage fluids
	Animals	Glomerular immune injury	Kidneys
	Human	Gastric mucosa injury	Stomach
	Human	Psoriasis	Skin lesion
		Ulcerative colitis, Crohn's diseases	Colonic mucosa
	Mice	Lupus nephritis	Kidneys

Cysteinyl-leukotrienes (LTC_4 and LTD_4) cause renal vasoconstriction, induce mesangial cell contraction and proliferation, and stimulate the production of extracellular matrix proteins. In a mouse model of lupus nephritis, LT production, which is significantly increased, is proportional to the functional and histopathologic severity of the renal disease. In this model, receptor inhibition of cysteinyl-leukotrienes significantly improved renal hemodynamics [34]. In the rat model of nephrotoxic serum nephritis a specific LTD_4 receptor antagonist prevented deterioration of glomerular hemodynamics [240]. In passive Heymann nephritis LTD_4 was shown to be a mediator of proteinuria and glomerular hemodynamic abnormalities [241], and its inhibition markedly blunted proteinuria and reversed hemodynamic dysfunction. In a model of cyclosporine nephrotoxicity cysteinyl-leukotrienes were found to play a role in the pathogenesis of renal disorder, and blockade of their receptors prevented functional and structural derangement [242].

The involvement of the various leukotrienes in several pathologic states is summarized in Table 2.**4**.

5-LOX-inhibition

In many experimental models inhibition of leukotriene synthesis is associated with improvement of pathologic states. The biological properties of leukotrienes, together with their formation in a variety of diseases, suggest that 5-lipoxygenase inhibitors should have therapeutic potential in a range of allergic and inflammatory conditions, e.g. asthma, rheumatoid arthritis, ulcerative colitis, etc.

However, the search for selective 5-LOX inhibitors has been on the whole rather disappointing [236, 243]. 5-LOX inhibitors have been classified as redox inhibitors, iron-chelating inhibitors, competitive inhibitors of 5-LOX, and FLAP inhibitors.

Redox inhibitors

The active site of 5-LOX contains a nonheme iron, which is liganded by His-367, His-372, His-550, and the carboxy-terminal Ile-673. In the resting state the iron is in the ferrous form. Activation of 5-LOX by hydroperoxides oxidizes the iron into the ferric form, which allows the enzyme to enter the catalytic cycle. The nonheme iron center of 5-LOX cycles between the ferrous and ferric states during catalysis. 5-LOX and the related arachidonic acid metabolizing enzymes are susceptible to inhibition by compounds with low redox potentials. Thus, "redox inhibitors" generally show poor selectivity for 5-LOX relative to COX. Furthermore, despite displaying potent activity *in vitro*, they are often weak or inactive enzyme inhibitors *in vivo* when administered orally. Besides natural compounds, such as coumarins (e.g. esculetin) and flavonoids (e.g. cirsiliol), prototypes of this class are phenidone and BW 755 C. Other members include indazolinone derivatives that combine high selectivity for the 5-LOX pathway with potent *in vivo* effects [244]. *However, these "redox inhibitors" may readily interact with other biological redox systems, and one toxic consequence of these interactions is the formation of methemoglobin.*

Iron chelators

Inhibition of 5-LOX can also be obtained with iron chelators. One of the most powerful metal ligand groups is the hydroxamic acid moiety; hydroxamic acids, and their close derivatives N-hydroxyureas (zileuton; ABT-761) show modest (10–40fold) selectivity for the inhibition of 5-lipoxygenase versus cyclooxygenases [245, 246].

Zileuton significantly reduces allergen-induced nasal congestion. It selectively blocks leukotriene release in the nasal lavage fluids of patients with allergic rhinitis following challenge with specific allergens [247], but in other studies, such as in rheumatoid arthritis and ulcerative colitis, administration of this drug did not show any statistical difference to placebo [248–250].

The methoxyalkylthiazole ICI 211,965 is a potent inhibitor of 5-lipoxygenase and does not inhibit cyclooxygenases [251, 252]. The derivative ICID 2138 is at least ten times more potent (*ex vivo* ED_{50} for 5-lipoxygenase inhibition = 1 mg kg^{-1} after oral administration), and no inhibition of cyclooxygenases has been observed even at concentrations up to 20,000 times higher than those that inhibit 5-lipoxygenase [236].

Other, less potent 5-lipoxygenase inhibitors of this class include REV 5901 and WY 50,295 [236, 253].

FLAP inhibitors

MK-591, an inhibitor of FLAP (five-lipoxygenase activating protein), has been shown to decrease proteinuria by restoring glomerular size selectivity in patients with glomerulonephritis [254]. In another study in patients with ulcerative colitis this compound inhibited leukotriene biosynthesis, but its clinical efficacy was not significantly different from that of placebo [255].

All these studies seem to indicate that the use of 5-LOX inhibitors may represent an insufficient single therapeutic model in inflammatory diseases other than asthma, in which the anti-inflammatory and antibronchospastic effects of these drugs act synergistically.

Thus, the discovery of compounds that are able to inhibit both main metabolic pathways of arachidonic acid metabolism merits interest.

2.7 Lipoxins

Lipoxins (LXs), members of the prostanoid family, have a trihydroxytetraene structure and are both structurally and functionally unique among arachidonic-acid-derived bioactive products (see Figs. 2.**11** and 2.**12**). These compounds can be produced by transcellular biosynthetic pathways during cell-cell interactions [256]. Multiple biosynthetic routes can lead to LX generation. In human cell types two main pathways have been demonstrated:

- 15-LOX-initiated pathway
- 5-LOX-initiated pathway: the LTA_4 route

A third major pathway for LX biosynthesis has recently been uncovered, the:

- Aspirin-triggered 15-epi-lipoxins circuit.

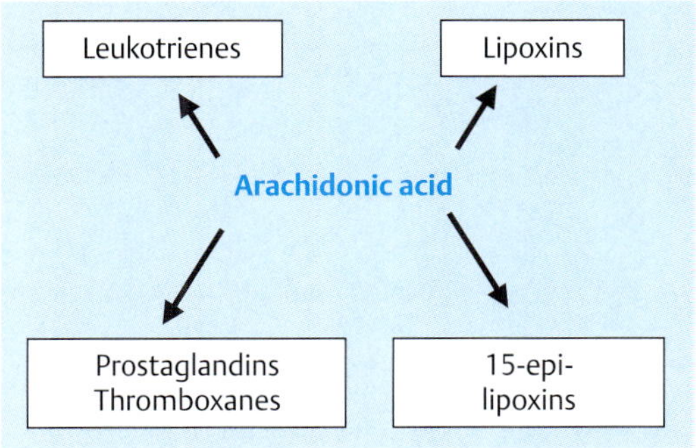

Fig. 2.**11** Lipoxins, arachidonic acid-derived bioactive products.

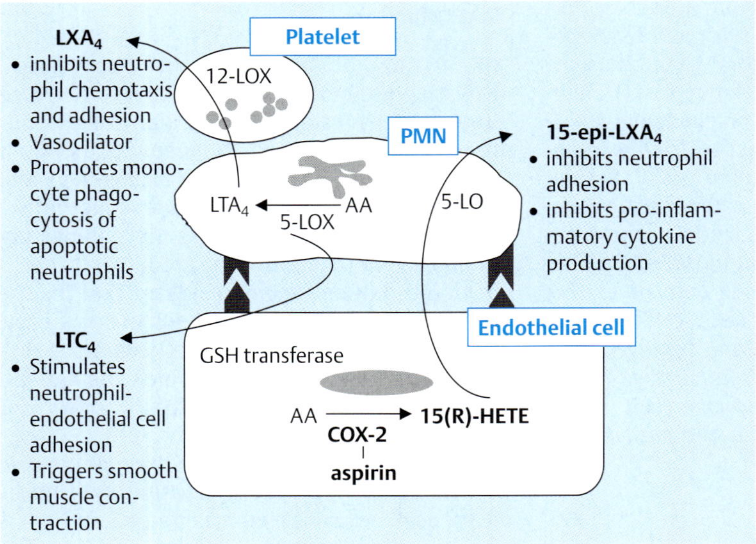

Fig. 2.**12** Transcellular biosynthesis of leukotriene, lipoxins and aspirin-triggered 15-epi-lipoxins.

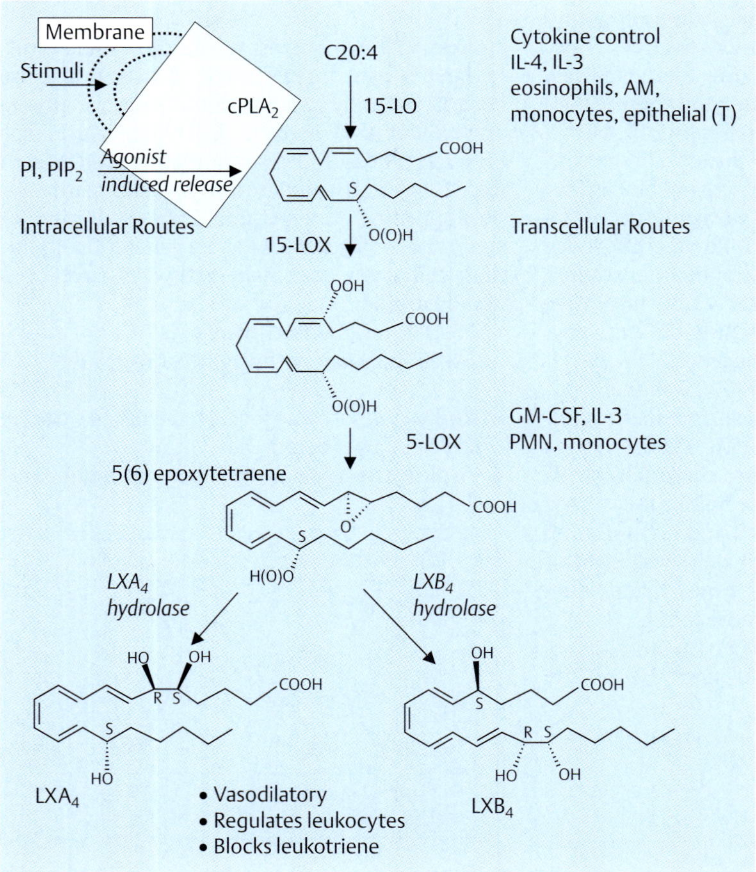

Fig. 2.**13** 15-LOX initiated LX biosynthesis.

15-LOX-initiated pathway

In this pathway (see Fig. 2.**13**) 15-LOX is involved in the generation of the bioactive molecules and inserts a molecular oxygen into the carbon 15 of the AA, predominantly in the *S* configuration, generating 15-HPETE and/or 15-HETE, compounds that can serve as substrates for 5-LOX. The product of the 5-lipoxygenase action on 15-HPETE is then rapidly converted to a 5,6-epoxytetraene, which can be rapidly converted to lipoxin A_4 (LXA_4) via LXA_4 hydrolase and/or via lipoxin B_4 hydrolase to lipoxin B_4 (LXB_4).

During the biosynthesis of lipoxins, leukotriene production is blocked at the 5-LOX level [257], generating an inverse relationship between leukotriene and lipoxin biosynthesis. Thus, when LXs are generated by neutrophils by conversion of 15-HETE, leukotriene formation is inhibited while LXs are released.

5-LOX- initiated pathway: the LTA_4 route

This recognized pathway for lipoxin biosynthesis occurs between cell types of the vasculature, which are usually blood-borne, for example, the interaction of human neutrophils with platelets (see Fig. 2.**14**). This biosynthetic system involves, as key oxygenases, 5-lipoxygenase within human neutrophils and 12-lipoxygenase, which is present in high amounts in human platelets (see Fig. 2.**14**) [258, 259]; it occurs predominantly within the vasculature when platelet glutathione is depleted and involves the 5-LOX-mediated release of LTA_4 from neutrophils and the subsequent conversion of this compound to LXs by platelets. In fact, neutrophils LTA_4 formed from 5-LOX and released to the extracellular milieu is picked up by PMN-adherent platelets. Platelet 12-lipoxygenase then abstracts a molecular hydrogen at carbon-13 and inserts a molecular oxygen into the carbon-15 of LTA_4, converting it to a carbonium cation intermediate that opens either to lipoxin B_4, when attacked by water at the carbon-14, or to lipoxin A_4, when attacked by water at carbon-6 [260–262]. The formation of both lipoxins, A_4 and B_4, is unique to platelet 12-LOX. This new activity of 12-LOX indicates that this enzyme serves as a lipoxin synthase in platelets. Indeed, the 12-lipoxygenase converts LTA_4 to LXs, A_4 and B_4. Of particular interest is the observation that 12-LOX undergoes suicide inactivation with LTA_4 as the substrate for LXB_4 but continues to generate LXA_4. This is thought to be a regulatory mechanism which may have implications for the biological actions of lipoxins A_4 and B_4 when generated within the vasculature, which is a likely site for platelets and leukocytes to adhere and interact [263, 264].

The 15-LOX-initiated pathway and the 5-LOX-initiated pathway/LTA_4 route are not inhibited by aspirin or aspirin-like drugs.

Aspirin-triggered 15-epi-lipoxins circuit

This third main pathway for lipoxin biosynthesis has been recently discovered [265, 266] (see Fig. 2.**15 a**). In this biosynthetic system COX-2 induced in either endothelial or epithelial cells via proinflammatory cytokines such as IL-1β, LPS or TNF switches its catalytic activity in the presence of aspirin, generating 15*R*-HETE. In this setting aspirin inhibits PG synthesis by both COX-1 and COX-2 [267] through irreversible acetylation, but while the acetylated form of COX-1 is not active, the aspirin-acetylated COX-2 remains active and converts endogenous arachidonic acid to 15*R*-HETE, which is then released and transformed via transcellular routes to form 15-epi-LXs by adherent leukocytes. The activated adherent leukocytes, which bear 5-LOX, transform 15*R*-HETE to a 5(6)-epoxytetraene, which also carries its C-15 alcohol group in the *R* configuration. This common intermediate leads to the formation of both, 15-epi-lipoxin A_4 and 15-epi-lipoxin B_4. 15-epi-lipoxin A_4 has proved to be more potent than LXA_4 in inhibiting neutrophil adhesion, and 15-epi-LXB_4 appears to be an inhibitor of cell proliferation [265]. Interest in this pathway derives from the fact that COX-2 is present in abundance in inflammatory reactions and in disease states [267–269] and is in place when individuals take aspirin for its therapeutic benefit. It is of particular interest to note that we have come to think of aspirin as an inhibitor of prostanoid synthesis, and these new results clearly establish that aspirin can trigger the biosynthesis of novel compounds, namely aspirin-triggered lipoxins (ATLs), which can serve as potential endogenous anti-inflammatory signals or mediators (see Fig. 2.**15 b**).

Tissues and disease: Lipoxins generation *in vivo*

The formation of native LXs has been demonstrated *in vivo* (see Table 2.**6**). Lipoxins are generated in human tissues, this first having been

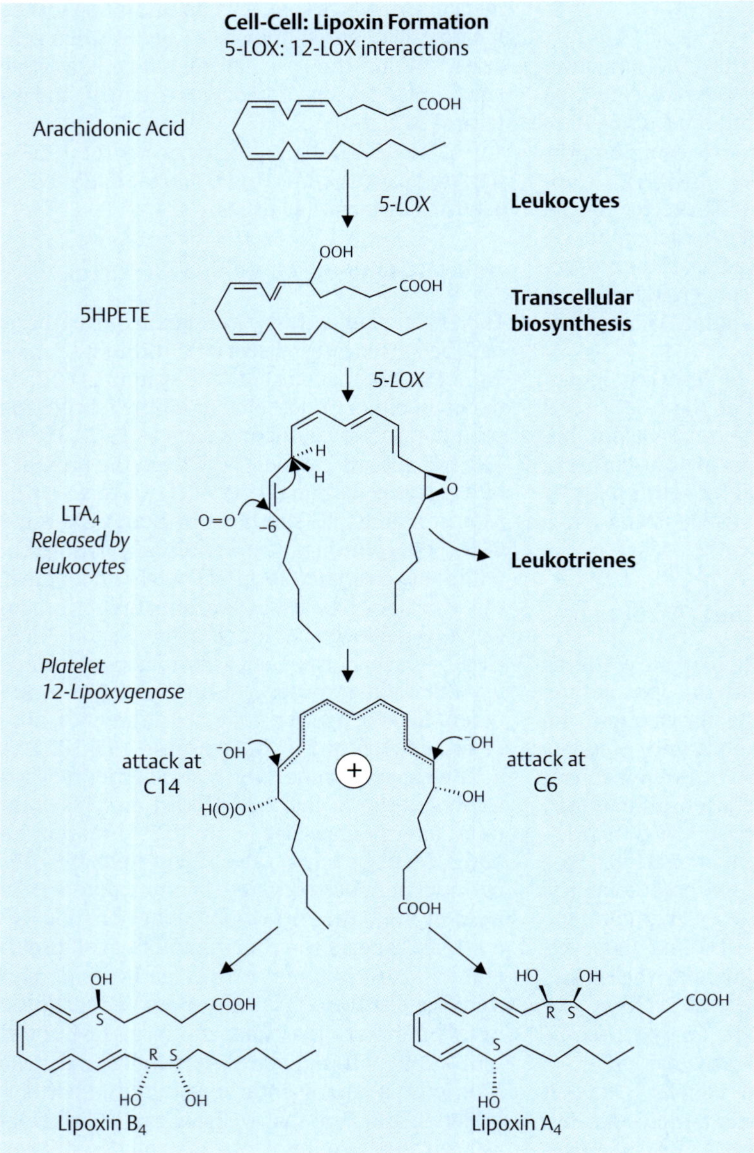

Fig. 2.**14** 5-LOX-12-LOX interactions in LX biosynthesis.

demonstrated in bronchoalveolar lavage fluids [270]. Lipoxins are formed in nasal polyps [270], and LXA_4 is generated in nasal lavage fluids from aspirin-sensitive asthmatics [270] and in experimental nephritis. In the intracoronary artery rupture of atherosclerotic plaque also leads to a rapid generation of lipoxin A_4 [270]. Lipoxins are also generated by activated whole blood *ex vivo* [270] and by normal human bone marrow [270]. During chronic myelocytic leukemia platelets lose 12-LOX as well as their ability to generate LXs. This finding may be related to the blast crisis observed in chronic myelocytic leukemia [270]. Recently it has been proposed that LXs are useful biomarkers for asthma [270] and for long-term clinical improvement in arthritic patients.

Some of the sites in which LXs have been demonstrated *in vivo* are summarized in Table 2.**5** [256].

The above list is not exhaustive and is likely to represent *in vivo* scenarios where cell-cell interaction is accelerated and the generation of LXs is

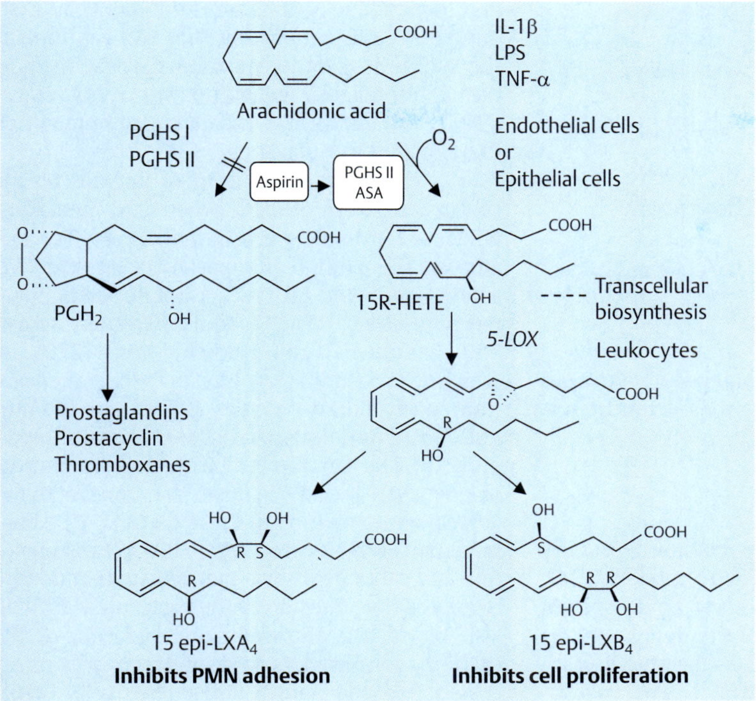

Fig. 2.**15** a Aspirin-triggered 15-epi-LX biosynthesis.

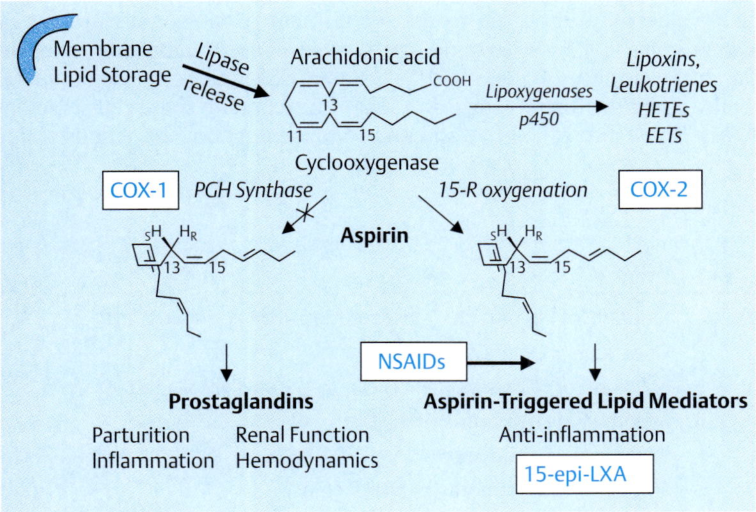

Fig. 2.**15 b** Aspirin-triggered lipoxin biosynthesis.

Table 2.**5** Tissues and disease: LX generation

Angioplastic-induced athero-sclerotic plaque rupture	Glomerulonephritis
Aspirin-sensitive asthmatics	Sarcoidosis
Asthma	Pneumonia
Normal bone marrow-defect in chronic myeloid leukemia	Nasal polyps
Activated whole blood	Rheumatoid arthritis

detected because of the abundance of cytokines and cell-cell interactions in these clinical settings.

Lipoxin functions

LXs display vasodilatory and counterregulatory roles in both *in vivo* and *in vitro* models [270]. They relax aorta and pulmonary arteries. LXA_4 can reverse precontraction of the pulmonary artery induced by $PGF_{2\alpha}$ as well as the potent vasoconstrictor enzyme endothelin-1. The mechanisms of LX-induced vasodilatation involves endothelium-dependent vasorelaxation, and both prostaglandin-dependent and prostaglandin-independent mechanisms. In some tissues lipoxins can stimulate the formation, for example, of prostacyclin by endothelial cells, which in turn can lead to vasodilatation [271]. These prostanoid-dependent actions are inhibitable by COX inhibitors [272], indicating that LXs can induce the synthesis of other mediators. These include the LX-stimulated generation of nitric oxide (NO) [270], which may mediate a component of LX-regulated vascular tone.

It is clear that the actions of lipoxins are in contrast to those of most other lipid mediators which are primarily pro-inflammatory. For example, LXA_4 exhibits human-leukocyte-selective actions (see Table 2.**6**), such as inhibition of polymorphonuclear (PMN) transmigration across both endothelial and epithelial cells [270], in which it is vasodilatory, blocks PMN diapedesis from postcapillary venules [270], and inhibits PMN entry into inflamed tissues in animal models [270]. LXs can also inhibit the transmigration of leukocytes by a mechanism that appears to involve downregulation of CD11/CD18 [270]. Thus, in human PMN LXs are likely to block transmigration and chemotaxis by a mechanism that downregulates the adhesion of the molecules [270]. It also blocks the intracellular generation of IP_3 [270]. By contrast, LXs have inhibitory actions on eosinophils and natural killer (NK) cells [270], and LXA_4 and LXB_4 stimulate chemotaxis and adherence in monocytes [270], which may be related to the recruitment of monocytes to sites of wound injury. In response to LXs, monocytes do not release superoxide anions or degranulate, suggesting that the action on these cells is selective and related to locomotion. The actions of lip-

Table 2.**6** Human-leukocyte-selective LX actions

	Leukocytes	Action
LXA_4	PMN	Blockade of emigration, transmigration and chemotaxis
		Downregulation of CD 11/18, IP_3, Ca^{2+}
		Inhibition of PMN-endothelial cells and epithelial cell interactions
	Eosinophils	Inhibition of chemotaxis (PAF, FMLP)
	NK cells	Inhibition of cytotoxicity
	Monocytes	Stimulation of chemotaxis and adherence
		Stimulation of myeloid progenitors
LXB_4	PMN	Blockade of emigration, transmigration and chemotaxis
		Downregulation of CD 11/18, IP_3, Ca^{2+}
		Inhibition of PMN-endothelial and epithelial cell interactions
	NK cells	Inhibition of cytotoxicity
	Monocytes	Stimulation of chemotaxis and adherence
		Stimulation of myeloid progenitors

Table 2.**7** Potential anti-inflammatory actions of LXs demonstrated *in vivo*

Lipoxin	Action
LXA_4	Inhibition of airway constriction in asthmatics
	Inhibition of PMN diapedesis from postcapillary venules
	Inhibition of PMN entry into inflamed renal tissue
	Regulation of LTB_4-mediated delayed hypersensitive reaction
	Antagonization of LTD_4-induced renal hemodynamics
LXB_4	Induction of sleep

oxins in these settings occur at subnanomolar concentrations.

LXs have also been shown to be potent stimuli for myeloid progenitors [270].

A potentially important role for LXA_4 in humans, is highlighted by the findings that LXA_4 administered by inhalation blocks airway constriction in asthmatics [270] (see Table 2.**7**). *In vivo*, LXs inhibit diapedesis of PMN from postcapillary venules [270] and inhibit the entry of leukocytes into inflamed tissues [284]. LXA_4 downregulates LTB_4-mediated delayed hypersensitive reactions [270], antagonizes the actions of LTD_4 in renal hemodynamics, and competes at the receptor for LTD_4 [270]. LXB_4 has been shown to induce sleep *in vivo*, a finding that has also been shown for PGD_2.

Hence, LXs not only provide counterregulatory roles in the physiologic events of inflammation but may also be actual effectors of well-established anti-inflammatory therapies.

LXs can act via one or a combination of three main mechanisms that depend in part on the cell type, and tissues concerned.

They can be illustrated as follows:

- LXs can act at their own cell surface receptors;
- LXA_4 interact with a subclass of LTD_4 receptors that also bind LXA_4;
- LXs can act at intracellular targets after LX transport/uptake or within its cell of origin [256].

2.8 Lipoxygenase/cyclooxygenase inhibition and related drugs

Considering that both prostaglandins and leukotrienes are involved in inflammatory processes, the inhibition of the pathways involved in arachidonic acid metabolism (COX and 5-LOX) could represent a strong therapeutic rationale in the development of new anti-inflammatory compounds (see Figs. 2.**16** and 2.**17**). Moreover, leukotriene synthesis may be increased by the inhibition of COX by NSAIDs, because in this case the arachidonic acid would be diverted to the 5-LOX pathway [273, 274]. Thus, it could be interesting to inhibit this pathway as well to avoid gastrointestinal and renal adverse effects. Drugs that are able to inhibit both COX and 5-LOX equally have been designed in order to obtain compounds that retain the activity of classical NSAIDs while avoiding their main drawbacks, i.e. the curtailed production of gastroprotective prostaglandins associated with the concurrent curtailed production of stomach-damaging and bronchoconstrictive leukotrienes. Moreover, as already seen, leukotrienes are pro-inflammatory; they increase microvascular permeability, are potent chemotactic agents, and attract eosinophils, neutrophils, and monocytes in the synovium [227, 275]. It is further advantageous for a compound to possess both activities, because prostaglandins enhance leukotriene-mediated inflammation [226, 276, 277].

Of course, it is in principle quite easy to design a drug that selectively acts on one enzyme. It is obviously a far more daunting task to design a drug that selectively inhibits two different enzymes. This is especially true if the two enzymes do not have a high degree of structural similarity. For any dual acting anti-inflammatory drug data should therefore be produced to show that COX and 5-LOX are indeed the only enzymes affected within a reasonably wide range of doses.

Moreover, attention should be paid to the possibility that prolonged inhibition of both the 5-LOX pathway and the COX pathway may cause side effects in long-term use.

Several chemically distinct compounds are currently in various phases of preclinical or clinical development, but none are commercially available, and no clinical study with these compounds has so far been published. However, animal studies have shown that these 5-LOX/COX inhibitors exert marked anti-inflammatory effects coupled with an almost complete lack of

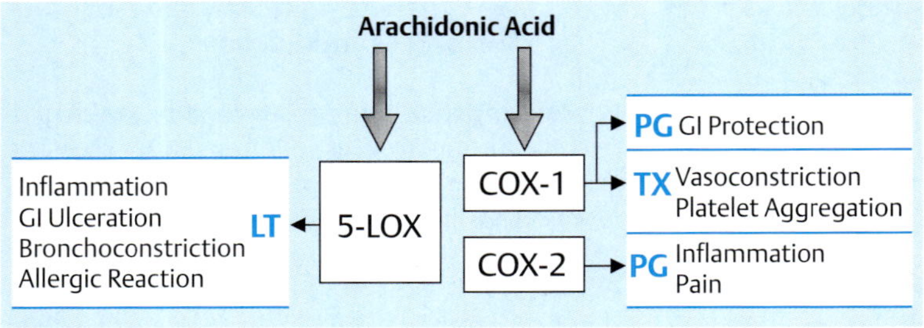

Fig. 2.**16** Pathways involved in the AA metabolism.

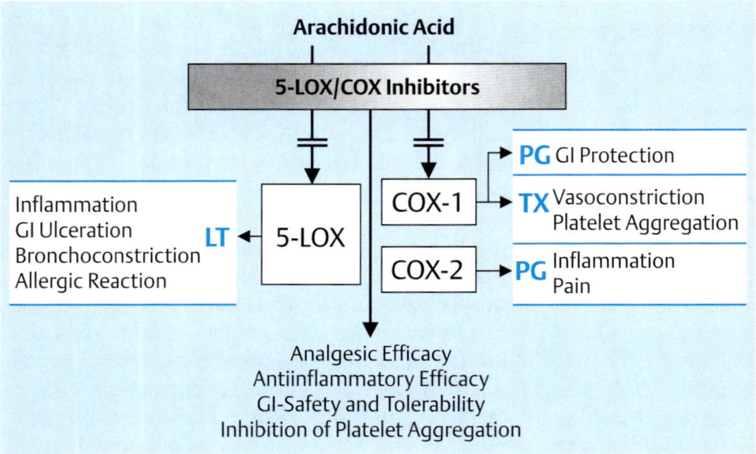

Fig. 2.**17** Inhibition of the pathways involved in the AA metabolism.

gastric toxicity. One of the first examples of a dual acting anti-inflammatory drug was tepoxalin [278, 279]. The IC_{50} of this compound for guinea-pig lung cyclooxygenase was found to be 0.80 µM, while the IC_{50} for cell-free 5-lipoxygenase was found to be 0.15 µM. The oral ED_{50} in adjuvant arthritis in rats – a well established standard model for predicting clinical antiarthritic efficacy – turned out to be 3 mg kg^{-1}. At single oral doses of 25 – 100 mg kg^{-1} in dogs **tepoxalin** inhibited the formation of PGE_2 and LTB_4 in synovial fluid from knee joints challenged with an intra-articular injection of sodium urate and rabbit anti-dog IgG immune complexes [277]. **Tepoxalin** was well tolerated at the gastric level in rats and dogs chronically treated for one and six months at doses several times higher than required for controlling inflammation [279, 280].

An important source of 5-LOX/COX inhibitors is the **di-tert-butylphenol class** of anti-inflammatory agents [281, 282]. Moreover, these compounds have antioxidant and radical scavenging properties which may contribute to their anti-inflammatory efficacy and low ulcerogenic potential [281].

Tebufelone was shown to be a competitive reversible inhibitor of COX with an IC_{50} of 1.5 µM [283]. It inhibited calcium ionophore-induced prostaglandin E_2 production by purified rat peritoneal macrophages with an IC_{50} of 0.02 µM, making it an order of magnitude more potent than indomethacin. **Tebufelone** also inhibited calcium ionophore-induced leukotriene B_4 production by rat macrophages with an IC_{50} of 20 µM and by human whole blood with an IC_{50} of 22 µM [283]. In human volunteers who received *Escherichia coli* endotoxin (2 ng kg^{-1} i.v.) as a pyrogen, **tebufelone** 50 mg exhibited antipyretic activity comparable to 650 mg of aspirin [284].

Another inhibitor of 5-LOX and COX-2 is **darbufelone** (CI 1004). *In vitro,* it inhibited COX-2 with an IC_{50} value of 0.48 µM but did not inhibit COX-1. In a randomized, double blind, escalating single- and multiple-dose study in healthy volunteers, it was well tolerated up to a daily oral dose of 100 mg [285, 286].

BF-389 was shown to have an oral ED_{50} in the adjuvant arthritis test in rats of 18 mg kg^{-1}/day (4 day-treatment). The ulcerogenic activity, evaluated in rats after a four-day treatment period, gave an oral UD50 of 520 mg kg^{-1}/day, the therapeutic ratio thus being 28. The IC_{50} for human leukocyte COX and 5-LOX were 0.84 and 3.65 µM, respectively [287].

RWJ 63,556 is a 5-LOX inhibitor which also possesses modest specific COX-2 inhibition. COX-2 was inhibited with an IC_{50} of 1.81 µM compared with > 10 µM for COX-1. Calcium ionophore-induced leukotriene B_4 production in isolated human peripheral blood leukocytes was inhibited with an IC_{50} value of 1.02 µM [288]. **RWJ 63,556,** 3 or 30 mg kg^{-1} per os once daily for 14 days in rats with adjuvant-induced arthritis reduced edema in the injected paw by 54% and 88.6%, respectively [289].

Another 5-LOX/COX inhibitor is PGV 20,229 [290]. This compound exhibited selectivity for COX-2 (human platelet COX-1, IC_{50} = 7 µM; human monocyte COX-2, IC_{50} = 0.22 µM) and inhibited leukotriene synthesis in RBI cells with an IC_{50} of 8 µM. **PGV 20,229** inhibited adjuvant arthritis in rats with an oral ED_{50} = 6.6 mg kg^{-1}.

2.9 Licofelone

Introduction

Traditional nonsteroidal anti-inflammatory drugs (NSAIDs) are among the most commonly used medications for the treatment of inflammatory disease [291]. They have anti-inflammatory, antipyretic, and analgesic properties and are prescribed as drugs of first choice for the treatment of rheumatic disorders and other joint diseases. The common mechanism of action of this class of drugs involves inhibition of the cyclooxygenase enzymes and consecutively the metabolism of arachidonic acid to inflammatory prostaglandins and thromboxane [292]. However, inhibition of the COX pathway by NSAIDs also reduces gastroprotective prostaglandin synthesis, resulting in the well-known gastrointestinal side effects which limit their use as anti-inflammatory drugs [292]. In addition, the resulting increase in leukotriene metabolites due to the shunting of arachidonic acid metabolism to the 5-lipoxygenase pathway causes additional gastrointestinal injury [293] (see Fig. 2.**18**). By inhibiting both cyclooxygenase and 5-lipoxygenase it should therefore be possible to develop compounds with reduced ulcerogenic side effects [292].

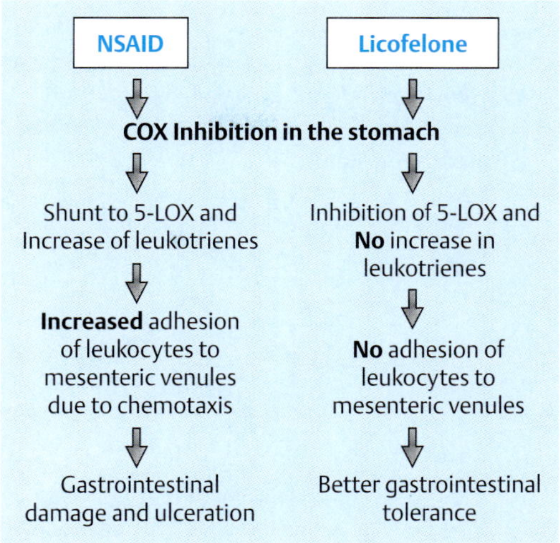

Fig. 2.**18** Shunting of arachidonic acid metabolism to the 5-lipoxygenase pathway.

In this section we will review the mechanism of action and pharmacodynamics of a promising new compound that has demonstrated both safety and efficacy in animal models and early clinical trials.

Among dual acting anti-inflammatory drugs, licofelone ([6-(4-chlorophenyl)-2,2-dimethyl-7-phenyl-2,3-dihydro-1 *H*-pyrrolizin-5-yl]acetic acid (see Fig. 2.**19**), previously called ML3000, a derivate of the phenyl moiety at the 6-position of the pyrrolizine ring, constitutes a novel class of nonantioxidant compound with a potent competitive (see Fig. 2.**20**) and well-balanced inhibitory effect on the COX and 5-LOX pathways (see Fig. 2.**21**). It is currently undergoing phase III clinical trials for the treatment of osteoarthritis [293–296]. This new pyrrolizine compound has analgesic, antipyretic, anti-inflammatory, anti-asthmatic, and antiplatelet aggregation activity at doses that do not cause gastrointestinal damage [297–299].

As mentioned above, it is a well-balanced dual inhibitor. In fact, it has been found to inhibit COX in bovine and human platelets with IC_{50} values of 0.16–0.21 µM and 5-LOX in bovine and human granulocytes with IC_{50} values of 0.18–0.23 µM, giving a COX/5-LOX ratio approaching 1 [298, 300].

In several models of analgesic (phenylquinone-induced writhing in mice, Randall-Selitto

Chemical name:
[6-(4-chlorophenyl)-2,2-dimethyl-7-phenyl-2,3-dihydro-1*H*-pyrrolizin-5-yl]acetic acid

Structural formula:

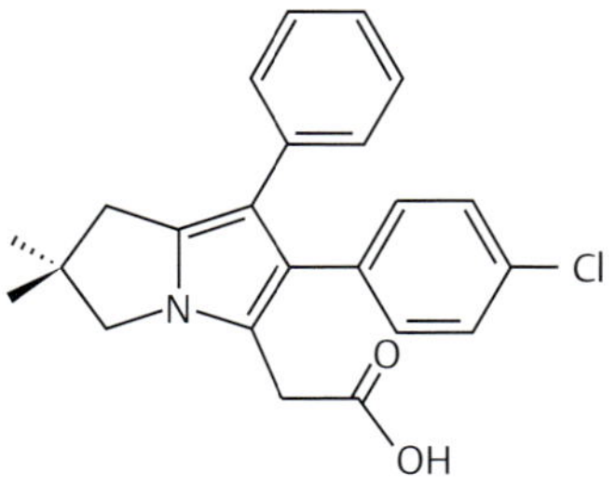

Fig. 2.**19** Chemical name and structural formula of licofelone.

assay in rats, etc.), anti-inflammatory (adjuvant arthritis in rats, carrageenan-induced rat paw edema, air pouch granuloma in rats, etc.), and antithrombotic (arachidonic-acid-induced rabbit and human platelet aggregation, laser-induced thrombus formation in rats, thromboembolism models in mice) activity, licofelone has been highly effective when given in oral doses of 10–100 mg/kg^{-1} [298, 300].

The anti-inflammatory activity has been mainly studied in the rat model of adjuvant arthritis. These models showed that the reduction of the experimentally induced secondary lesions and paw swelling obtained with licofelone was similar to that seen with indomethacin [299] and that the compound can reduce synovial cell proliferation, histological damage, and joint erosions in an affected ankle joint [301]. The effects of licofelone on experimentally induced cartilage lesions were also studied in a dog model (osteoarthritis was induced by anterior cruciate ligament section); compared with placebo, licofelone significantly reduced the size and grade of erosions and histological damage [302] by exerting an inhibitory effect on PGE_2 in synovial fluid and on local LTB_4 production.

This compound has exhibited a favorable tissue distribution pattern, with highest tested levels being reached in the lungs, liver, kidneys, heart, and large and small intestines [303].

Oral administration of licofelone at doses of 30–300 mg/kg in rats produced no gastrointestinal damage [297].

Orally administered licofelone exhibited potent antiasthmatic activity (ED_{50} = 0.2–12 mg kg^{-1} i.v.) in guinea-pigs challenged with arachidonic acid or antigen and in sheep challenged with antigen [297, 298].

Mechanism of action

Effect on prostaglandin and leukotriene production

The effects of licofelone on the production of prostanoids were evaluated using a series of cellular test systems and *in vivo* experiments demonstrating the activity of licofelone in specific tissues [304]. In a single dose of 10, 30, and 100 mg/kg compared to indomethacin at 10 mg/kg and in the vehicle-control carrageenan-induced rat paw edema model licofelone exhibited complete inhibition of both PGE_2 and LTB_4 secretion at all dose levels, while indomethacin exhibited complete inhibition of PGE_2 only [304]. These data confirm previous findings in the carrageenan-in-

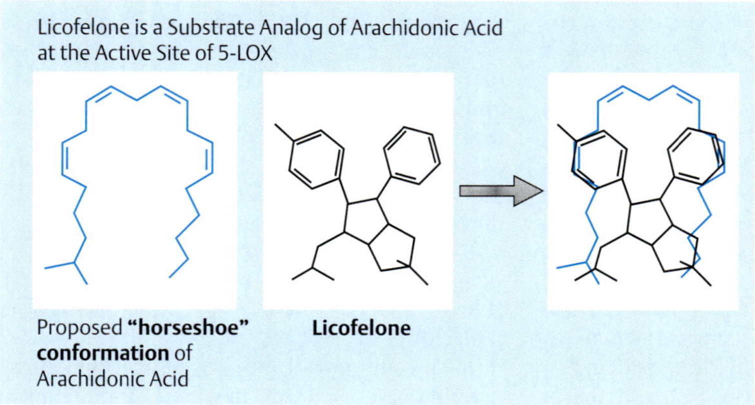

Fig. 2.**20** Licofelone chemical structure.

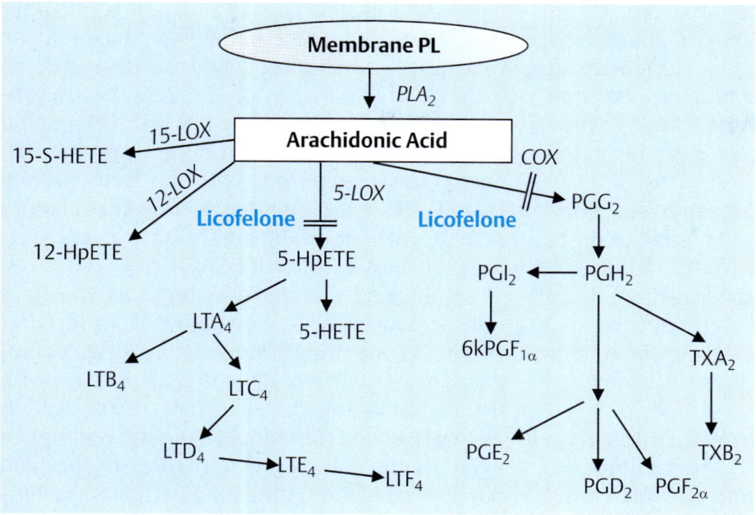

Fig. 2.**21** Licofelone mechanism of action.

duced rat paw edema model, where the ED_{50} of licofelone for oral administration was 17 mg/kg versus 3 mg/kg for indomethacin. While indomethacin was more potent in this experimental model of inflammation, licofelone produced significantly less gastric injury. In fact, the ulcerogenic dose (UD_{50}) for indomethacin was 7 mg/kg, while licofelone was tolerated well up to the highest dose tested (100 mg/kg p.o.) [299]. The enhanced formation of leukotriene metabolites during treatment with NSAIDs in the inflamed tissue appeared to play a key role in the development of adverse effects of these drugs in the respiratory and gastrointestinal tract [305, 306]. Peptidoleukotrienes and LTB_4 increases have been reported to play an important pathophysiologic role in the induction of gastrointestinal ulceration [298, 307]. The inhibition of leukotrienes by licofelone in colonic tissue was evaluated in a trinitrobenzenesulfonic acid-induced colonic inflammation study in rats. This study showed that a single oral dose of licofelone 10 mg/kg inhibited the synthesis of LTB_4 as effectively as a single dose of MK-886 10 mg/kg, a known leukotriene inhibitor [304]. In the same paper the authors compared the effects of licofelone, diclofenac, and indomethacin on the production of PGE_2 and LTB_4 in the stomach, using a rat *ex vivo* model. PGE_2 production in the stomach was significantly inhibited by diclofenac (1 and 3 mg/kg), indomethacin (0.3, 1, and 3 mg/kg), and licofelone (10, 30, 100 mg/kg) at the doses tested. But licofelone caused no increased generation of detrimental LTB_4 in the rat stomach, while diclofenac and indomethacin induced a significant increase of LTB_4 levels. This finding suggests that traditional NSAIDs, while blocking the production of pro-inflammatory prostaglandins, also create a shunt to the 5-LOX pathway that results in increased production of leukotrienes. It also demonstrates the mechanism of the gastric-sparing properties of licofelone.

To further demonstrate the 5-LOX inhibitory action of licofelone, the effects of intragastric administration of licofelone on leukocyte adherence to postcapillary mesenteric venules in rats were compared to the effects of indomethacin and control. The extent of leukocyte adherence was determined at 30, 60, 90, and 120 minutes. Indomethacin 20 mg/kg caused significant adherence at 60, 90, and 120 min., whereas licofelone 3 and 100 mg/kg did not cause significant adherence, compared to control [293]. The inhibition of LTB_4 by licofelone was also shown in basophilic leukemia cells (RBL-1 cells), a common model for the investigation of 5-LOX metabolites. Licofelone inhibited LTB_4 generation with an IC_{50} value of 3.6 µM. For NDGA, a very potent antioxidant suppressor of LTB_4 production, an IC_{50} value of the same order of magnitude (2.15 µM) was calculated [304].

Anti-LOX activity and novel activities

In another *in vitro* study [308] the anti-LOX activity of licofelone was confirmed, and an inhibitory effect on the production of 5-LOX metabolites generated as a consequence of platelet-PMN transcellular metabolism was observed. In the same work new activities of the compound were identified, e.g. its ability to block superoxide anion generation, lysosomal granule secretion, and Mac-1-mediated homotypic PMN aggregation, three of the most relevant PMN responses to inflammatory agonists.

These experiments extend the previous observation that licofelone inhibits LT production by leukocytes, indicating the ability of the drug to interfere with the enzymatic activity of 5-LOX inside the cell and to inhibit LT production in a mixed cell system in which PMN cooperate with platelets in the generation of these inflammatory mediators.

At concentrations lower than 10 µM licofelone inhibited the formation of LTA_4-derived metabolites including LTB_4, the nonenzymatic derivative 6- and 12-*trans*-LTB_4, and the transcellular metabolite LTC_4 and enhanced the production of the mixed 5 and 12-LOX product, 5,12-diHETE. These results indicate that, in the low concentration range, the drug selectively blocks the 5-LOX activity that converts 5-HPETE to LTA_4, shifting AA metabolism toward the formation of 5-HPETE. At higher concentrations licofelone inhibits all 5-LOX activity.

In addition to the effect on LT synthesis, licofelone inhibited the generation of superoxide anions, the release of elastase, and the increased expression of the β2 integrin Mac-1 on the PMN surface. At comparable concentrations it also inhibited Mac-1-dependent PMN homotypic PMN aggregation. Licofelone may therefore also interfere with the signaling pathway switched on by the G-protein-coupled receptor of fMLP that leads to the activation of Mac-1 independently of its anti-LOX and anti-COX activities. The anti-adhesive property of ML3000 appears to depend on the effect of the drug on a cellular target distinct from 5-LOX or COX.

Thus, licofelone not only interferes with oxidative and secretory processes in activated PMN but also with the functional activation of the β2 integrin required for competent binding to its counterreceptors [308].

Anti-inflammatory activity

Studies in carrageenan-induced paw edema and adjuvant arthritis models demonstrated that licofelone is an active anti-inflammatory compound. In the carrageenan-induced paw edema model, licofelone showed an ED_{50} of 17 mg/kg p.o. with a plasma concentration of about 20 µ/ml. Although indomethacin was shown to be four times as active as licofelone with an ED_{50} of 3 mg/kg, it also had a UD_{50} of 7 mg/kg. By contrast, in licofelone-treated rats the UD_{50} could not be calculated due to the high gastric tolerance at the doses tested [293]. This study showed that licofelone has significant anti-inflammatory activity without producing the gastric injury often seen with traditional NSAIDs.

Significant anti-inflammatory activity was also demonstrated in two adjuvant arthritis rat studies. In one study groups of ten rats with adjuvant arthritis were orally dosed for 28 days with licofelone 80 mg/kg, licofelone 80 mg/kg or 20 mg/kg and acetaminophen, or acetaminophen alone. Erythema and edema scores of the hind paw recorded during the 28-day treatment period were statistically lower in the group receiving licofelone 20 mg/kg and acetaminophen than in the group receiving only acetaminophen. No difference was seen between the licofelone 80 mg/kg plus paracetamol and the licofelone 80 mg/kg without acetaminophen groups. Histopathologic examinations of knee and ankle joints showed that licofelone had an anti-inflammatory and antidestructive effect at both doses, 20 mg/kg and 80 mg/kg, compared to control [293].

In another adjuvant arthritis rat model groups of ten rats were orally dosed b.i.d. with licofelone 10 mg/kg, licofelone 25 mg/kg, licofelone 50 mg/kg, or indomethacin 1.0 mg/kg. Twenty rats were dosed with vehicle b.i.d. Adjuvant arthritis was induced on day 2. From day 10 onwards the secondary lesions on the uninjected paws, ears, and tail were scored subjectively. Decreases in secondary lesions in rats treated with licofelone 25 mg/kg were similar to the decreases seen with indomethacin. Injected paw volumes in rats treated with licofelone 10 mg/kg p.o. or higher dosages were similar to volumes in indomethacin-treated rats [293]. In these animal models the anti-inflammatory activity of licofelone was comparable to that of indomethacin.

Analgesic activity

The analgesic effects of licofelone were demonstrated in two animal models. Phenylquinone writhing is used as a screening model to evaluate the analgesic activity of peripherally and centrally acting compounds. Licofelone 10 mg/kg p.o. was more effective than aspirin 50 mg/kg p.o. on phenylquinone writhing in mice [293]. In the

Randall and Selitto assay oral administration of peripherally active analgesics, such as NSAIDs, enhances the pain threshold of inflamed paws in rats. Licofelone 30 mg/kg was as effective as indomethacin 10 mg/kg in increasing pain threshold of inflamed paws in rats at 0.5, 1, 2, and 3 hours following administration [293].

Antipyretic activity

Licofelone showed antipyretic activity in brewer's yeast-induced hyperthermia in the rat. A significant antipyretic effect was seen with licofelone 10 mg/kg p.o. that lasted over three hours and was comparable to the effect of indomethacin 10 mg/kg p.o. [293].

Anti-asthmatic activity

Anti-asthmatic activity of licofelone was demonstrated in three animal models. Licofelone inhibited bronchoconstriction in the guinea pig arachidonic acid-induced bronchoconstriction model with an ED_{50} 0.2 ± 0.05 after intravenous administration. In a similar guinea pig model, oral licofelone 100 mg/kg showed the same activity as indomethacin 10 mg/kg [293].

Licofelone also exhibited anti-asthmatic activity in the antigen-induced bronchoconstriction model in guinea pigs. In this model the ED_{50} for licofelone was 12.3 ± 1.0 mg/kg i.v., while the reference drugs, phenidone at 30 mg/kg i.v. and NDG at 10 mg/kg i.v., produced 80% and 52% inhibition, respectively, of transpulmonary pressure increase [293]. Licofelone's COX and 5-LOX inhibitory activity and anti-asthmatic activity were further demonstrated in the sheep asthma model, since both COX and 5-LOX metabolites are key components of the endpoints of this model. Licofelone 100 mg/sheep, delivered by aerosol, significantly reduced early airway response and significantly inhibited late airway response in seven sheep [293]. Results of this study suggest that aerosol administration of a balanced inhibitor of COX and 5-LOX may have beneficial effects in the treatment of allergic airway disease.

The activity of licofelone as a balanced inhibitor of both cyclooxygenase and 5-lipoxygenase is shown by its ability to inhibit bronchoconstriction in these animal models.

Antiaggregating and antithrombotic activity

Licofelone has significant antithrombotic activity in *in vivo* animal models in comparison to aspirin and inhibits platelet aggregation in human plasma using different inducers [298, 309].

In a recent paper [309] the platelet antiaggregating activity of licofelone was shown to reduce thrombus formation in an *in vivo* laser-induced thrombosis model. A significant dose-dependent increase in the number of laser lesions needed to induce thrombus formation in the mesenteric vessels of rats was seen with licofelone at 10, 30, and 100 mg/kg p.o. The antithrombotic activity of licofelone was comparable to that of aspirin, and the effect lasted up to 12 hours postadministration. The antithrombotic and antiaggregating activity of licofelone is very interesting; in fact, this drug maintains these activities like the nonselective NSAIDs but it is safer for the GI tract than the selective COX-2 inhibitors, which, as mentioned, do not provide protection against the risk of a thrombotic event and even increase such risk in patients with cardiovascular problems.

Gastrointestinal tolerability

A single-dose and a repeated-dose animal study have shown excellent gastrointestinal tolerability for licofelone [292, 295]. Groups of five rats each were given indomethacin (5, 10, or 20 mg/kg), licofelone (3, 10, 30, or 100 mg/kg) or vehicle orally. Three hours later the rats were killed and the stomach was removed. Any macroscopically visible lesions were measured and a gastric damage score was calculated. In this study, while indomethacin caused significant injury to the gastric mucosa characterized by hemorrhagic bands at all the doses tested, licofelone did not induce injury at any of the doses tested that differed significantly from that observed in the vehicle-treated controls. This study also showed that licofelone caused dose-dependent inhibition of prostaglandin E_2 synthesis by the stomach and by the blood at the highest dose tested (100 mg/kg) and at the doses in the 30 – 100 mg/kg range, respectively, comparable to that seen with indomethacin at 20 mg/kg. Also, after oral administration of licofelone (100 mg/kg), gastric LTB_4 synthesis was not significantly different from that measured in rats treated with vehicle. In terms of leukocyte adherence to postcapillary mesenteric venules, indomethacin caused profound leukocyte adherence, while licofelone did not cause significant leukocyte adherence at any of the doses tested [295].

In treatment groups of ten rats each single oral administration of licofelone at doses of 10, 30, 100 mg/kg produced no gastric or duodenal damage, while a single oral dose of 10 mg/kg indomethacin produced marked and statistically significant gastric and duodenal damage in all the treated animals. Repeated oral administration of licofelone at daily doses of 10, 30, 100 mg/kg produced only slight intestinal damage, but the effect was minimal and was not found to be statistically significant. Licofelone was clearly better tolerated by the gastrointestinal tract than indomethacin, which at doses of 3 mg/kg p.o. caused significant gastric and duodenal damage, such as mucosal necrosis and bleeding [292]. Moreover, licofelone administered repeatedly to rabbits produced no gastric damage, while diclofenac, a widely used NSAID, produced penetrating antral ulcers in 64% of the animals [295], The studies described above demonstrate the differences in gastrointestinal tolerability between licofelone and traditional NSAIDs, suggesting that inhibition of the 5-lipooxygenase pathway could explain the gastric-sparing properties of this dual inhibitor (see Fig. 2.**18**).

A clinical study by Fiorucci et al. [310] investigated whether licofelone spares the gastric mucosa in aspirin-treated rats. Rats were treated orally for two weeks with 50 mg/kg/day aspirin and were then given placebo, licofelone (10, 30, and 100 mg/kg), or celecoxib (30 mg/kg). Rats were sacrificed six hours after the last dose, and gastric damage scores were determined and myeloperoxidase (MPO) activity measured. Gastric COX-1, COX-0,2 and 5-LOX expression was assessed by RT-PCR. Aspirin resulted in a significant increase in the damage score, 90% reduction of PGE_2 and TBX_2 levels, but increased COX-2 expression in the gastric mucosa. Celecoxib alone caused no gastric damage but worsened gastric mucosal damage in aspirin-treated rats. Licofelone alone spared the gastric mucosa and did not aggravate mucosal damage in aspirin-treated rats.

Beside its ability to inhibit COX-1 and COX-2, aspirin triggers the formation of potent bioactive lipoxins (15-epi-LXA_4) that may contribute to the therapeutic effect of this drug. Aspirin-triggered 15-epi-LXA_4 biosynthesis is initiated by acetylation of COX-2. This study provided evidence that gastric adaptation to aspirin is associated with increased COX-2 expression in the gastric mucosa and 15-epi-LXA_4 generation. Inhibition of 15-epi-LXA_4 production by selective and nonselective COX inhibitors (celecoxib, indomethacin, and ketoprofen) reverses mucosal adaptation to aspirin. By contrast, inhibition of 5-LOX and leukotriene formation with a dual inhibitor or a 5-selective inhibitor rescues the mucosa from damage induced by the administration of COX-inhibitors to aspirin-treated rats, indicating that a balance between 5-LOX products and aspirin-triggered 15-epi-LXA_4, is essential for gastric mucosal adaptation to aspirin [310].

Slowing of the progression of OA

Increased cartilage degradation and secondary synovitis are key events in the pathogenesis of OA, and it appears that the synovitis is fundamental to the appearance and progression of cartilage lesions [223]. This is due in part to the secretion of proinflammatory mediators that increase cartilage catabolism. Among these factors are interleukin-1β and tumor necrosis factor-α, which are present and elaborated in OA joint tissues. These cytokines have been shown to suppress the synthesis of cartilage matrix macromolecules while stimulating extracellular matrix destructive metalloproteases [223]. LTB_4, which has been detected in significant quantities in the synovial fluid and joint tissues of untreated control animals with OA, has been shown to be a potent factor in stimulating the synthesis of these cytokines [311]. Furthermore, treatment with chemical inhibitors of LOX, FLAP, and/or LTA_4 hydrolase was found to inhibit the severity of the disease [311].

In an experimental osteoarthritis dog model [311] licofelone administered twice daily at oral doses of 2.5 mg/kg/day and 5 mg/kg/day, significantly decreased the size and grade of cartilage lesions on the condyles and tibial plateaus of both groups treated compared to placebo. At the histological level the severity of the cartilage lesions was also decreased in the licofelone-treated dogs versus placebo-treated dogs in both, condyles and plateaus. Moreover, licofelone significantly reduced the level of PGE_2 in the synovial fluid and synovial LTB_4 production and markedly reduced levels of collagenase-1 and IL-1β, catabolic factors which, as discussed earlier, are known to play an important role in the pathophysiology of OA lesions. Licofelone has therefore been shown to significantly reduce the progression of lesions in experimental OA in dogs.

Chondrocyte apoptosis

Based on recent studies on the pathophysiology of OA, the loss of cartilage matrix, one of the most characteristic morphological changes associated with OA, is related to several factors leading to an imbalance in synthetic and degradative processes [312]. Today the role of proinflammatory cytokines and nitric oxide appears preponderant [312]. However, an additional factor recently proposed is the death of chondrocytes by the common phenomena known as apoptosis, which is accentuated by the loss of matrix [312].

The chondrocyte death/apoptotic phenomena in OA is complex and appears to be related to the excess synthesis of factors having pro-apoptotic activity in cartilage and synovium, among which NO and PGE_2 appear to dominate [312].

In a canine ligament transection model of OA [312] licofelone at oral doses of 2.5 mg/kg/day and 5 mg/kg/day markedly reduced the level of chondrocyte apoptosis and significantly decreased the levels of caspase-3, COX-2, and inducible NO in cartilage from both condyles and plateaus compared to the control (placebo) group. Licofelone is therefore an effective treatment *in vivo*, capable of reducing the level of OA chondrocyte death that is probably mediated by a reduction in the level of caspase-3 activity, which, in turn, may be related to the reduced production of two factors involved in the chondrocyte apoptosis, NO and PGE_2.

Clinical experience

Phase I. A pain study carried out with healthy human volunteers showed that a single oral dose of licofelone (200 or 400 mg) produced comparable analgesia to that achieved with ibuprofen at 800 mg, with analgesic effects evident within 35 to 40 minutes of administration [294]. In addition, phase I trials of licofelone have also shown a very good kinetic profile of the drug without any significant side-effects [294].

Phase II. Initial phase II results have confirmed the activity of licofelone and shown it to be well tolerated in osteoarthritis (OA). In a phase IIb double-blind trial in OA of the knee 100, 200 and 400 mg doses of licofelone b.i.d., were all significantly more effective than placebo and the response was dose related. Endpoints in this study were the Western Ontario and McMaster Universities (WOMAC) osteoarthritis index as a global score, with pain, stiffness and disability used as subscores. No serious adverse events were observed at any of the doses tested [294, 296].

The excellent GI safety observed in preclinical studies was confirmed in a four-week gastroscopy study in healthy volunteers who received licofelone 200 and 400 mg b.i.d., naproxen 500 mg b.i.d., or placebo. Naproxen showed significant toxicity, while the licofelone results were very similar to those observed with placebo. Endpoints of this study were posttreatment Lanza scores [296].

Conclusions

In summary, licofelone is a novel, potent, balanced, competitive inhibitor of both COXs and 5-LOX with demonstrated anti-inflammatory, analgesic, antipyretic, antiasthmatic, and antiplatelet aggregation activity in several animal models. It has proven activity and has shown excellent gastrointestinal tolerability in both animal experiments and in phase I and II clinical trials. Licofelone is now undergoing phase III testing.

2.10 References

1 Wittcoff H. The Phosphatides. New York: Rheinhold Press, 1951: 99
2 Chang J, Musser JH, McGregor H. Phospholipase A_2: function and pharmacological regulation. Biochem Pharmacol 1987; 36: 2429 – 2436
3 Dennis EA. Diversity of group types, regulation and function of phospholipase A_2. J Biol Chem 1994; 269: 13,057 – 13,060
4 Six DA, Dennis EA. The expanding superfamily of phospholipase A_2 enzymes: classification and characterisation. Biochim Biophys Acta. 2000; 1488: 1 – 19
5 Whinkler JD et al. Biochemical and pharmacological comparison of cytosolic, high molecular weight phospholipase A_2, human synovial fluid phospholipase A_2 and CaO-independent transacyclase. J. Lipid Mediators cell signal. 1994; 10: 315 – 330
6 Dennis EA. The growing phospholipase A_2 superfamily of signal transduction enzymes. Trends Biochem Sci 1997; 22: 1 – 2
7 Fitzpatrick FA, Soberman R. Regulated formation of eicosanoids. J Clin Invest 2001; 107: 1347 – 1351
8 Vadas P, Browning J, Edelson J, Pruzanski W. Extracellular phospholipase A_2 expression and inflammation: the relationship with associated disease states. J Lip Mediat 1993; 8: 1 – 309
9 Dan P, Nitzan DW, Dagan A, Ginsburg I, Yedgar S. H_2O_2 renders cells accessible to lysis by exogenous phospholipase A_2: a novel mechanism for cell damage in inflammatory processes. FEBS Lett 1996; 383: 75 – 78

[10] Kundu GC, Mukerjee AB. Evidence that porcine pancreatic phospholipase A_2 via its high affinity receptor stimulates extracellular matrix invasion by normal and cancer cells J Biol Chem 1997; 272: 2346–2353

[11] Denizot Y, Dubery C, Desplat V, Praloran V. Incorporation and effect of arachidonic acid on the growth of the human K562 cell line. Cancer Lett 1999; 139: 75–78

[12] Balsinde J, Balboa MA, Insel PA, Dennis EA. Regulation and inhibition of phospholipase A_2. Annu Rev Pharmacol Toxicol 1999; 39: 175–189

[13] Parente L. Pros and cons of selective inhibition of cyclooxygenase-2 versus dual lipoxygenase/cyclooxygenase inhibition. Is two better than one? J Rheumatol 2001; 28: 2375–2382

[14] Smith WL, Garavito RM, DeWitt DL. Prostaglandin endoperoxide H synthases (cyclooxygenase)-1 and –2. J Biol Chem 1996; 271: 33,157–33,160

[15] Fu JY, Masferrer JL, Seibert K, Needleman P. The induction and suppression of prostaglandin H_2 synthase in human monocytes. J Biol Chem 1990; 265: 16,737–16,740

[16] Xie WL, Chipman JG, Robertson DL, Simmons DL. Expression of a nitrogen-responsiveness gene encoding prostaglandin synthase is regulated by mRNA splicing. Proc Natl Acad Sci USA 1991; 88: 2692–2696

[17] Kujubu DA, Fletcher BS, Varnum BC, Lim RW, Herschman HR. TIS10, a phorbol ester tumour promoter-inducible mRNA from Swiss 3T3 cells, encodes a novel prostaglandin synthase/cyclooxygenase homologue. J Biol Chem 1991; 266: 12,866–12,872

[18] Celotti F, Laufer S. Anti-inflammatory drugs: new multitarget compounds to face an old problem. The dual inhibition concept. Pharmacol Research. 2001; 43: 429–436

[19] Bertolini A, Otani A, Sandrini M. Dual acting anti-inflammatory drugs: a reappraisal. Pharmacol Res 2001; 43: 1–14

[20] Kurumbail RG, Stevens AM, Gierse JK, McDonald JJ, Stegeman RA, Pak JK et al. Structural basis for selective inhibition of cyclooxygenase-2 by anti-inflammatory agents. Nature 1996; 384: 644–648

[21] Luong C, Miller A, Barnett J, Chow J, Ramesa C, Browner MF et al. Flexibility of the NSAID binding site in the structure of human cyclooxygenase-2. Nature Struct Biol 1996; 3: 927–933

[22] Picot D, Loll PJ, Garavito M. The X-ray crystal structure of the membrane protein prostaglandin H_2 synthase. Nature 1994; 367: 243–249

[23] Garavito RM. The three-dimensional structure of cyclooxygenases. In: Vane J, Botting J, Botting R (eds). Improved non-steroid anti-inflammatory drugs: COX-2 enzyme inhibitors. Dordrecht: Kluwer Academic Publishers, 1996: 29–43

[24] Hawkey C. COX-2 inhibitors. Lancet 1999; 353: 307–314

[25] Wong E, Bayly C, Waterman HL, Riendeau D, Mancini JA. Conversion of prostaglandin G/H synthase-1 into an enzyme sensitive to PGHS-2 selective inhibitor by a double His513 to Arg nd Ile523 to Val mutation. J Biol Chem 1997; 272: 9280–9286

[26] Lanzo CA, Beechmen JM, Talley J, Marnett LJ. Investigation of the binding of isoform selective inhibitors to endoperoxide synthase using fluorescence spectroscopy. Biochemistry 1998; 37: 217–226

[27] Marnett LJ, Kalgutkar A. Cyclooxygenase-2 inhibitors: discovery and future. TIPS 1999; 20: 465–469

[28] Spencer AG, Woods JW, Arakawa T, Singer II, Smith WL. Subcellular localization of prostaglandin endoperoxide H synthase-1 and -2 by immunoelectron microscopy. J Biol Chem 1998; 273: 9886–9893

[29] Bozza PT, Yu WG, Penrose JF, Morgan ES, Dvorak AM, Weller PF. Eosinophil lipid bodies: specific, inducible intracellular sites for enhanced eicosanoids formation. J Exp Med 1997; 186: 909–920

[30] Crofford L. COX-1 and COX-2 tissue expression: implication and predictions. J Reumatol 1997; 24 (Suppl 49): 15–19

[31] Lipsky PE. Role of Cyclooxygenase-1 and -2 in health and disease. Am J Orthop 1999; 28 (Suppl 3): 8–12

[32] Sigal E. The molecular biology of mammalian arachidonic acid metabolism. Am J Physiol 1991; 260: L13-L28

[33] Langenbach R, Morham SG, Tiano HF, Loftin CD, Ghanayem BI, Chulada PC et al. Disruption of the mouse cyclooxygenase-1 gene. Characteristics of the mutant and areas of future study. Adv Exp Med Biol 1997; 407: 87–92

[34] Langenbach R, Loftin CD, Lee C, Tiano HF. Cyclooxygenase knockout mice: models for elucidating isoform-specific functions. Biochem Pharmacol 1999; 58: 1237–1246

[35] Langenbach R, Loftin CD, Lee C, Tiano H. Cyclooxygenase-deficient mice. A summary of their characteristics and susceptibilities to inflammation and carcinogenesis. Ann N Y Acad Sci 1999; 889: 52–61

[36] Smith, WL, Langen Bach R. Why there are two cyclooxygenase isozymes. J Clinical Invest 2001; 107: 1491–1495

[37] Sugimoto Y, Narumiya S, Ichikawa A. Distribution and function of prostanoid receptors: studies on knockout mice. Prog Lipid Res 2000; 39: 289–314

[38] Patrignani P et al. Biochemical and pharmacological characterisation of the cyclooxygenase activity of human blood prostaglandin endoperoxide synthase. J Pharmacol Exp Ther 1994; 271: 1705–1712

[39] Langenbach R, Morham SG, Tiano HF, Loftin CD, Ghanayem BI, Chulada PC, Mahler JF, Lee CA, Goulding EH, Kim HS, Smithies C. Prostaglandin synthase 1 gene disruption in mice reduces arachidonic acid-induced inflammation and indomethacin-induced gastric ulceration. Cell 1995; 83: 483–492

[40] Patrono C. Prevention of myocardial infarction and stroke by aspirin: different dosage? Throm Res 1998; 92: S7–S12

[41] Lim H et al. Multiple female reproductive failures in cyclooxygenase-2-deficient mice. Cell 1997; 91: 197–208

[42] Gross G et al. Opposing actions of prostaglandins and oxytocin determine the onset of murine labour. Proc Natl Acad Sci USA 1998; 95: 11,875 – 11,879
[43] Gross G et al. Inhibition of cyclooxygenase-2 prevents inflammation-mediated preterm labour in the mouse. Am J Physiol Regul Integr Comp Physiol 2000; 278: R1415-R1423
[44] Dinchuck JE et al. Renal abnormalities and an altered inflammatory response in mine lacking cyclooxygenase-2. Nature 1995; 378: 406 – 409
[45] Davis BJ et al. Anovulation in cyclooxygenase-2-deficient mice is restored by prostaglandin E_2 and interleukin-1 beta. Endocrinology 1999; 140: 2685 – 2695
[46] Lim H et al. Cyclooxygenase-2-derived prostacylin mediates embryo implantation in the mouse via PPAR delta. Genes Dev 1999; 13: 1561 – 1574
[47] Komhoff M et al. Cyclooxygenase-2 selective inhibitors impair glomerulogenesis and renal cortical development. Kidney Int 2000; 57: 414 – 422
[48] Loftin CD et al. Failure of ductus arterious closure and remodelling in neonatal mice deficient in cyclooxygenase-1 and -2. Proc Natl Acad Sci USA 2001; 98: 1059 – 1064
[49] Morham SG, Langenbach R, Loftin CD, Jennette JC, Tiano HF, Mahler JH, Ledford A, Lee CA, Smithies O. Prostaglandin synthase-2-gene disruption causes severe renal pathology in the mouse. Cell 1995; 83: 473 – 448
[50] Dinchuck JE et al. Renal abnormalities and an altered inflammatory response in mine lacking cyclooxygenase-2. Nature 1995; 378: 406 – 409
[51] Wallace JL, Bak A, McKnight W, Asafha S, Sharka KA, MacNaughton WK. Cyclooxygenase-1 contributes to inflammatory responses in rats and mice: implications for gastrointestinal toxicity. Gastroenterology 1998; 115: 101 – 109
[52] Gilroy DW, Colville-Nash PR, Willis D, Chivers J, Willoughby DA. Inducible cyclooxygenase may have anti-inflammatory properties. Nat Med 1999; 5: 698 – 701
[53] Tatsuguchi A et al. Localization of cyclooxygenase-1 and ayclooxygenase-2 in Helicobacter pylori related gastritis and gastric tissues in humans. Gut 2000; 46: 782 – 789
[54] Austin SC, Funk CD. Insight into prostaglandin, leukotriene and other eicosanoid functions using mice with targeted gene disruptions. Prostaglandins Lipid Mediat 1999; 58: 231 – 252
[55] Lipsky PE, Brooks P, Crofford LJ, DuBois R, Graham D, Simon S et al. Unresolved issues in the role of cyclooxygenase-2 in normal physiologic processes and disease. Arch Intern Med 2000; 160: 913 – 920
[56] Wallace JL. Selective COX-2 inhibitors: is the water becoming muddy? Trends Pharmacol Sci 2001; 20: 4 – 6
[57] Mizuno H et al. Induction of cyclooxygenase-2 in gastric mucosal lesions and its inhibition by specific antagonist delays healing in mice. Gastroenterology 1997; 112: 387 – 397
[58] Shmassmann A et al. Effects of inhibition of prostaglandin endoperoxide synthase-2 in chronic gastrointestinal ulcer models in rats. Br J Pharmacol 1998; 123: 795 – 804
[59] Tsujii M et al. Cyclooxygenase regulates angiogenesis induced by colon cancer cells. Cell 1998; 93: 705 – 716
[60] Hull MA et al. Expression of basic fibroblast growth factor in intact and ulcerated human gastric mucosa. Gut 1998; 43: 525 – 536
[61] Jackson ML et al. COX-1 expression in human gastric mucosa infected with Helicobacter pylori: constitutive or induced? Gastroenterology 1998; 114: A160
[62] McLaughlan J et al. Increased inducible cyclooxygenase associated with treatment failure in ulcerative colitis. Gastroenterology 1996; 110: A964
[63] Wallace JL et al. NSAID-induced damage in rats: requirement of both cyclooxygenase-1 and -2. Gastroenterology 2000; 119: 706 – 714
[64] Zimmermann KC et al. Constitutive cyclooxygenase-2 expression in healthy human and rabbit gastric mucosa. Mol Pharmacol 1998; 54: 536 – 540
[65] Chulada PC et al. Genetic distruption of Ptgs-1, as well as Ptgs-2, reduces intestinal tumorgenesis in Min mice. Cancer Res 2000; 60: 4705 – 4708
[66] Houchon CW et al. Disruption of the cyclooxygenase-1 gene results in an impaired response to radiation injury. Am J Pathol 2000; 279: G858-G865
[67] Prescott SM, White RL. Self-promotion?. Intimate connection between APC and prostaglandin H synthase-2. Cell 1996; 87: 783 – 786
[68] Jacoby RF et al. The COX-2 inhibitor celecoxib is a potent preventive and therapeutic agent in the Min mouse model of adenomatous polyposis. Cancer Res 2000; 60: 5040 – 5044
[69] Souza RF et al. Selective inhibition of cyclooxygenase-2 suppresses growth and induces apoptosis in human esophageal adenocarcinoma cells. Cancer Res 2000; 60: 5767 – 5772
[70] Prescott SM, White RL. Self promotion? Intimate connections between APC and prostaglandin H synthase-2. Cell 1996; 87: 783 – 786
[71] Spencer AG, Woods JW, Arakawa T, Singer II, Smith W. Subcellular localization of prostaglandin endoperoxide H synthases-1 and -2 by immunoelectron microscopy. J Biol Chem 1998; 273: 9886 – 9893
[72] Smith WL, Dewitt DL, Garavito RM. Cyclooxygenases: structural, cellular and molecular biology. Annu Rev Biochem 2000; 69: 149 – 182
[73] Shitashige M, Morita I, Murota S. Different substrate utilisation between prostaglandin endoperoxide H synthase-1 and – 2 in NIH3T3 fibroblasts. Biochem Biophys Acta 1998; 1389: 57 – 66
[74] Murakami M, Kambe T, Shimbara S, Kudo I. Functional coupling between various phospholipase A_2s and cyclooxygenases in immediate and delayed prostanoid biosynthetic pathways. J Biol Chem 1999; 274: 3103 – 3115
[75] Chen W, Pawelek TR, Kulmacz RJ. Hydroperoxide dependence and co-operative cyclooxygenase kinetics

in prostaglandin H synthase-1 and -2. J Biol Chem 1999; 274: 20,301 – 20,306
[76] Swinney DC et al. Differential allosteric regulation of prostaglandin H synthase 1 and 2 by arachidonic acid. J Biol Chem 1997; 272: 12,393 – 12,398
[77] Murakami M et al. Regulation of prostaglandin E_2 biosynthesis by inducible membrane-associated prostaglandin E_2 synthase that acts in concert with cyclooxygenase-2. J Biol Chem 2000; 275: 32,783 – 32,792
[78] Fitzpatrick FA, Soberman R. Regulated formation of eicosanoids. J Clin Invest 2001; 107: 1347 – 1351
[79] Murakami M et al. Regulation of prostaglandin E_2 biosynthesis by inducible membrane-associated prostaglandin E_2 synthase that acts in concert with cyclooxygenase-2. J Biol Chem 2000; 275: 32,783 – 32,792
[80] TaniokaT, Nakatami Y, Semmyo N, Murakami M, Kudo I. Molecular identification of cytosolic prostaglandin E_2 synthase that is functionally coupled with cyclooxygenase-1 in immediate prostaglandin E_2 biosynthesis. J Biol Chem 2000; 275: 32,775 – 32,782
[81] Murakami M et al. Functional coupling between various phospholipase A_2s and cyclooxygenases in immediate and delate prostanoids biosynthetic pathways. J Biol Chem 1999; 274: 3103 – 3115
[82] Bezzini S et al. Exogenously added human group X secreted phospholipase A(2) but not the group IB, IIA, and V enzymes efficiently release arachidonic acid from adherent mammalian cells. J Biol Chem 2000; 275: 3179 – 3191
[83] Gijon MA et al. Cytosolic phospholipase A_2 is required for macrophage arachidonic acid release by agonists that do and do not mobilize calcium. Novel role of mitogen-activated protein kinase pathways in cytosolic phospholipase A_2 regulation. J Biol Chem 2000; 275: 20,146 – 20,156
[84] Balsinde J, Balboa MA, Dennis EA. Identification of a third pathway for arachidonic acid mobilisation and prostaglandin production in activated P388D1 macrophage-like cells. J Biol Chem 2000; 275: 22,544 – 22,549
[85] Coleman RA, Smith WL, Narumiya S. International Union of Pharmacology classification of prostanoid receptors: properties, distribution, and structure of the receptors and their subtypes. Pharmacol Rev 1994; 46: 205 – 229
[86] Narumiya S, Sugimoto Y, Ushikubi F. Prostanoid receptor, structure, properties, and functions. Physiol Rev 1999; 79: 1193 – 1226
[87] Halushka PV, Mais DE, Mayeux PR, Morinelli TA. Thromboxane, prostaglandin and leukotriene receptors. Annu Rev Pharmacol Toxicol 1989; 29: 213 – 219
[88] Coleman R, Smith WL, Narumiya S. International Union of Pharmacology classification of prostanoid receptors: properties, distribution and structure of the receptors and their subtypes. Pharmacol Rev 1994; 46: 205 – 229
[89] Forman BM, Tontonoz P, Chen J, Brun RP, Spiegelman BM, Evans RM. 15-Deoxy-delta 12,14-prostaglandin J2 is a ligand for adipocyte determination factor PPAR gamma. Cell 1995; 83: 803 – 812
[90] Lehmann JM, Lenhard JM, Oliver BB, Ringold GM, Kliewer SA. Peroxisome proliferator-activated receptors alfa and gamma are activated by indomethacin and other non-steroidal anti-inflammatory drugs. J Biol Chem 1997; 272: 3406 – 3410
[91] Ricote M, Li AC, Wilson TM, Kelly CJ, Glass CK. The peroxisome proliferator-activated receptors gamma is a negative regulator of macrophage activation. Nature 1998; 391: 79 – 82
[92] Colville-Nash PR, Qureshi SS, Willis D, Willoughby DA. Inhibition of inducible nitric oxide synthase by peroxisome proliferator-activated receptors agonists: correlation with induction of heme oxygenase 1. J Immunol 1998; 161: 978 – 984
[93] Jang C, Ting AT, Seed B. PPAR gamma agonists inhibit production of monocyte inflammatory cytokines. Nature 1998; 391: 82 – 86
[94] Jakobsson PJ, Thoren S, Morgenstern R, Samuelsson B. Identification of human prostaglandin E synthase: a microsomal, glutathione-dependent, inducible, enzyme, constituting a potent novel drug target. Proc Natl Acad Sci USA 1999; 96: 7220 – 7225
[95] Naraba H, Murakami M, Matsumoto H, Shimbara S, Ueno A, Kudo I et al. Segregated coupling of PLA2, cyclooxygenases and terminal prostanoid synthases in different phases of prostanoid biosynthesis in rat peritoneal macrophages. J Immunol 1998; 160: 2974 – 2982
[96] Brock T, McNish R, Peters-Golden M. Arachidonic acid is preferentially metabolised by cyclooxygenase-2 to prostacyclin and prostaglandin E2. J Biol Chem 1999; 274: 11,660 – 11,666
[97] Kudo I, Tanioka T, Nakatani Y, Semnyo N, Naraba H, Ueno A et al. Identification of two distinct PGE2 synthases that display different functional coupling with two cyclooxygenases. Abstract 11th International Conference on Advances in Prostaglandin, Leukotriene Research. Florence, Italy June 4 – 8, 2000: 23
[98] Kuchinde W, Barski O, Watanabe K, Hayaishi O. A long type prostaglandin F synthase is expressed in bovine liver: cDNA sequence and expression in E. coli. Biochem Biophys Res Commun 1992; 183: 1236 – 1246
[99] Suzuki-Yamamoto T, Nishizawa M, Fukiu M, Okuda-Ashitaka E, Nakajima T, Ito S et al. cDNA cloning, expression, and characterization of human prostaglandin F synthase. FEBS Lett 1999; 462: 335 – 340
[100] Chen LY, Watanabe K, Hayashi O. Purification and characterization of prostaglandin F synthase from bovine liver. Arch Biochem Biophys 1992; 296: 17 – 26
[101] Urade K, Watanabe K, Hayaishi O. Prostaglandin D, E, F synthases. J Lipid Mediat Cell Signal 1995; 12: 257 – 273

[102] Nusing R, Schneider-Voss S, Ullrich V. Immunoaffinity purification of human thromboxane synthase. Arch Biochem Biophys 1990; 280: 325–330
[103] Yokoyama C, Miyata A, Ihara H, Ullrich V, Tanabe T. Molecular cloning of human platelet thromboxane A synthase. Biochem Biophys Res Commun 1991; 178: 1479–1484
[104] Smith WL, DeWitt DL, Allen ML. Bimodal distribution of the prostaglandin I_2 synthase antigen in smooth muscle cells. J Biol Chem 1983; 258: 5922–5926
[105] Moncada S, Vane JR. Pharmacology and endogenous roles of prostaglandin endoperoxides, thromboxane A_2 and protacyclin. Pharmacol Rev 1978; 30: 293–331
[106] Austin, SC, Funk CD. Insight into prostaglandin, leukotriene, and other eicosanoid functions using mice with targeted gene disruptions. Prostaglandins Other Lipid Mediators 1999; 58: 231–252
[107] Hardy CC et al. The bronchoconstrictor effect of inhaled prostaglandin D_2 in normal and asthmatic men. N Eng J Med 1984; 311: 210–213
[108] Fuller RW et al. Prostaglandin D_2 potentiates airway responses to histamine and methacholine. Am Rev Resp Dis 1986; 133: 252–254
[109] Barnes PJ. Cytokines as mediators of chronic asthma. Am J Respir Crit Care Med 1994; 150: S42–49
[110] Mitchell JA, Larkin S, Williams TJ. Cyclooxygenase-2: regulation and relevance in inflammation. Biochem Pharmacol 1995; 50: 1535–1542
[111] Newton R et al. Evidence for the involvement of NFκB in the transcriptional control of cyclooxygenase-2 gene expression by interleukine-1β. Biochem Biophys Res Commun. 1997; 237: 28–32
[112] Springall DR et al. Inflammatory genes in asthmatic airway epithelium: suppression by corticosteroids. Eur Resp J 1995: 8 (Suppl 19): 44 S
[113] Frossard N, Stretton CD, Barnes PJ. Modulation of bradykinine responses in airway smooth muscle by epithelial enzymes. Agents Actions 1990; 31: 204–209
[114] Frossard N, Rhoden KJ, Barnes PJ. Influence of epithelium on guinea pig airway responses to tachykinins: role of endopeptidase and cyclooxygenase. J Pharmacol Exp Ther 1989; 248: 292–298
[115] Devillier P et al. Respiratory epithelium releases relaxant prostaglandin E_2 through activation of substance P (NK_1) receptors. Am Rev Resp Dis 1991; 139: A351
[116] Battistini B, Filep J, Sirois P. Potent thromboxane-mediated in vitro bronchoconstrictor effect of endothelin in guinea pig. Eur J Pharmacol 1990; 178: 141–142
[117] Goldie RG et al. Airway epithelium-derived inhibitory factor. Trends Pharmacol Sci 1990; 11: 67–70
[118] Pavord ID, Tattersfield AE. Bronchoprotective role for endogenous prostaglandin E_2. Lancet 1995; 344: 436–438
[119] Szczeklik A. Aspirin-induced asthma as a viral disease. Clin Allergy 1988; 18: 15–20
[120] Szczeklik A. Prostaglandin E and aspirin-induced asthma. Lancet 1995; 345: 1056
[121] Kuitert LM et al. Eicosanoid mediator expression in mononuclear and polymorphonuclear cells in normal subjects and patients with atopic asthma and cystic fibrosis. Thorax 1996; 51: 1223–1228
[122] Farman N, Pradelles P, Bonvalet JP. PGE_2, $PGF_{2\alpha}$, 6-keto-$PGF_{1\alpha}$ and TXB_2 synthesis along the rabbit nephron. Am J Physiol 1987; 252: F53–F59
[123] Ferreira SH. Prostaglandins, aspirin-like drugs and analgesia. Nature 1972; 240: 200–203
[124] Cao C et al. Cyclooxygenase-2 is induced in brain blood vessels during fever evoked by peripheral or central administration of tumor necrosis factor. Mol Brain Res 1998; 56: 45–56
[125] Higgs EA et al. Inflammatory effects of prostacyclin (PGI_2) and 6-oxo-$PGF_{1\alpha}$ in the rat paw. Prostaglandins 1978; 16: 153–162
[126] Pablos JL et al. Cyclooxygenase-1 and –2 are expressed by human T cells. Clin Exp Immunol 1999; 115: 86–90
[127] Kunkel SL, Chensus SW, Phan SH. Prostaglandins as endogenous mediators of interleukin 1 production. J Immunol 1986; 136: 186–192
[128] Kunkel SL et al. Regulation of macrophage tumour necrosis factor production by prostaglandin E_2. Biochem Biophys Res Commun 1986; 137: 404–410
[129] Kunkel SL et al. Prostaglandin E_2 regulates macrophage-derived tumor necrosis factor gene expression. J Biol Chem 1988; 263: 5380–5384
[130] Parker CW. Leukotrienes and prostaglandins in the immune system. Adv Prostaglandin Thromboxane Leukotriene Res 1986; 16: 113–134
[131] Desa FM et al. The effect of indometachin in the cartilage breakdown. Agents Actions 1989; 27: 485–487
[132] Pettipher ER et al. Indometachin enhances proteoglycan loss from articular cartilage in antigen-induced arthritis. Br J Pharmacol 1988; 94: 341 P
[133] Johansson C, Kollberg B. Stimulation by intragastrically administered E_2 prostaglandins of human gastric mucus output. Eur J Pharmacol 1979; 9: 229–232
[134] Allen A, Garner A. Mucus and bicarbonate secretion in the stomach and their possible role in mucosal protection. Gut 1980; 21: 249–262
[135] Bahari HMM, Ross IN, Tunberg LA. Demonstration of a gradient across the mucus layer on the surface of human gastric mucosa in vitro. Gut 1982; 23: 513–516
[136] Yamagata K et al. Expression of a mitogen-inducible cyclooxygenase in brain neurons; regulation by synaptic activity and glucocorticoids. Neuron 1993; 11: 371–386
[137] Breder CD, Dewitt D, Kraig RP. Characterisation of inducible cyclooxygenase in rat brain. J Comp Neurol 1995; 355: 296–315
[138] Cao C et al. Induction by lipopolysaccharide of cyclooxygenase-2 mRNA in rat brain; its possible

role in the febrile response. Brain Res 1995; 697: 187 – 196
[139] Ogorochi T et al. Regional distribution of prostaglandin D_2, E_2 and $F_{2\alpha}$ and related enzymes in postmortem human brain. J Neurochem 1984; 43: 71 – 92
[140] Narumiya S et al. Prostaglandin D_2 in rat brain, spinal cord and pituitary: basal levels and regional distribution. Life Sci 1982; 31: 2093 – 2103
[141] Ueno R et al. Prostaglandin D_2 induces sleep when microinjected into the preoptic area of conscious rats. Biochem Biophys Res Commun 1982; 109: 576 – 582
[142] Hayaishi O. Molecular mechanisms of sleep-wake regulation: roles of prostaglandins D_2 and E_2. FASEB J 1991, 5: 2575 – 2581
[143] Ueno R et al. Role of prostaglandin D_2 in the hyperthermia of rats caused by bacterial lipopolysaccharide. Proc Natl Acad Sci USA 1982; 79: 6093 – 6097
[144] Milton AS, Wendlandt S. Effects on body temperature of prostaglandins of the A, E and F series on injection into the third ventricle of unanaesthetised cats and rabbits. J Physiol (Lond) 1971; 218: 325 – 326
[145] Shapiro SS. Treatment of dysmenorrhoea and premenstrual syndrome with non-steroidal anti-inflammatory drugs. Drugs 1988; 36: 475 – 490
[146] Roberts LJ II, Oates JA. Biochemical diagnosis of systemic mast cells disorders. J Invest Dermatol 1991; 96: 19 S – 25 S
[147] Metcalf DD. The treatment of mastocytosis: an overview. J Invest Dermatol 1991; 96: 55 S – 59 S
[148] Brenner DE, Harvey HA, Lipton A, Demers L. A study of prostaglandin E_2, parathormone, and response to indometachin in patients with hypercalcemia of malignancy. Cancer 1982; 49: 556 – 561
[149] Gupta RA, DuBois RN. Aspirin, NSAIDs, and colon cancer prevention: mechanisms?. Gatroenterology 1998; 114: 1095 – 1098
[150] Symposium (various authors). Nonsteroidal anti-inflammatory drug-induced gastrointestinal damage. Current insight into patient management. Proceedings of a Symposium, June 13, 1987, Washington, D. C. Am J Med 1988 a; 84: 1 – 52
[151] Brater DC. Effects of nonsteroidal anti-inflammatory drugs on renal function: focus on cyclooxygenase-2-selective inhibition. Am J Med 1999; 107: 65 S – 70 S
[152] Whelton A. Renal and related cardiovascular effects of conventional and COX-2-specific NSAIDs and non-NSAID analgesics. Am J Ther 2000; 7: 63 – 74
[153] Clarkson MR et al. Leukotrienes and lipoxins: lipoxygenase-derived modulators of leukocyte recruitment and vascular tone in glomerulonephritis. Nephrol Dial Transplant 1998; 13: 3043 – 3051
[154] Lianos EA, Bresnahan BA. Effect of thromboxane A_2 inhibition and antagonism on prostaglandin and leukotriene synthesis in glomerular immune injury. J Lab Clin Med 1999; 134: 478 – 482
[155] McAdam BF et al. Systemic biosynthesis of prostacyclin by cyclooxygenase (COX)-2: the human pharmacology of a selective inhibitor of COX-2. Proct Natl Acad Sci USA 1999; 96: 272 – 277
[156] Pairet M, Van Ryn J, Mauz A, Scheirok H, Diederen W. Differential inhibition of COX1 and COX2 by NSAIDs: a summary of results obtained using various test systems. In: Vane JR, Botting J (eds). Selective Cyclooxygenase-2 Inhibitors: Pharmacology, Clinical Effects and Therapeutic Potential. Dordrecht: Kluwer Academic Publishers, 1998: 27 – 46
[157] Tavares IA, Bishai PM, Bennet PM. Activity of nimesulide on inducible cyclooxygenase. Arzneim-Forsch/Drug Res 1995; 45: 1093 – 1095
[158] Noble S, Balfor JA. Meloxicam. Drugs 1996; 51: 424 – 432
[159] Patrignani P, Panara MR, Sciulli MG, Santini G, Renda G, Patrono C. Differential inhibition of human prostaglandin endoperoxide synthase-1 and – 2 by nonsteroidal anti-inflammatory drugs. Physiol Pharmacol 1997; 48: 623 – 631
[160] Glaser K, Sund ML, O'Neil K. Etodolac selectively inhibits human prostaglandin G/H synthase 2 (PGHS-2) versus human PGHS-1. Eur J Pharmacol 1995; 281: 107 – 111
[161] Hallyar J, Bjanson I. NSAIDs, COX2 inhibitors, and the gut. Lancet 1995; 346: 521 – 522
[162] Cipollone F, Ganci A, Panara MR, Greco A, Cuccurullo F, Patrono C. Effect of nabumetone on prostanoidsynthesis in humans. Clin Pharmacol Ther 1995; 58: 335 – 341
[163] Van Ryn J, Pairet M. Selective cyclooxygenase-2 inhibitors: pharmacology, clinical effects and therapeutic potential. Drugs 1997; 6: 609 – 614
[164] Brooks P, Emery P, Evans JF, Fenner H, Hawkey CJ, Patrono C, Smolen J, Breedveld F, Day R, Dougados M, Ehrich EW, Gijon-Banos J, Kvien TK, van Rijswijk MH, Warner T, Zeidler H. Interpreting the clinical significance of differential inhibition of cyclooxygenase-1 and cyclooxygenase-2. Rheumatology 1999; 38: 779 – 788
[165] Isakson P, Zweifel B, Masferrer J. Specific COX-2 inhibitors: from bench to bedside. In: Vane JR, Botting J (eds). Selective cyclooxygenase-2 Inhibitors: Pharmacology, Clinical Effects and Therapeutic Potential. London: William Havery Press, 1997: 127 – 133
[166] Lipsky PE, Isakson P. Outcome of specific COX-2 inhibition in rheumatoid arthritis. J Rheumatol 1997; 24: 9 – 14
[167] Silverstein FE, Faich G, Goldstein JL et al. Gastrointestinal toxicity with celecoxib vs nonsteroidal anti-inflammatory drugs for osteoarthritis and rheumatoid arthritis. The CLASS study: a randomised controlled trial. JAMA 2000; 284: 1247 – 1255
[168] McAdam RF, Catella-Lawson F, Nardini IA, Fitzgerald GA. Systemic biosynthesis of prostacyclin cyclooxygenase (COX)-2: the human pharmacology of a selective inhibitor of COX-2. Proc Natl Acad Sci USA 1999; 96: 272 – 277

[169] Scott LJ, Lamb HM. Rofecoxib. Drugs 1999; 58: 499 – 505

[170] Lanza FL, Rack MF, Callison DA. A pilot endoscopic study of gastroduodenal effects of SC58635, a novel COX-2 inhibitor. Gastroenterology 1997; 112: A194

[171] Warner TD, Giuliano F, Vojnovic I, Bukasa A, Mitchell JA, Vane JH. Nonsteroidal drug selectivities for cyclooxygenase-1 rather than cyclooxygenase-2 are associated with human gastrointestinal toxicity: a full in vitro analysis. Proc Natl Acad Sci USA 1999; 96: 7563 – 7568

[172] Ehrich EW, Dallob A, DeLepeleire I. Characterisation of rofecoxib as a cyclooxygenase-2-isoform inhibitor and demonstration of analgesia in the dental pain model. Clin Pharmacol Ther 1999; 65: 336 – 347

[173] Cannon G, Caldwell J, Holt P. MK-0966, a specific COX-2 inhibitor has clinical efficacy comparable to diclofenac in the treatment of knee and hip osteoarthritis in 26-week controlled clinical trial. Arthritis Rheum 1998; 41: S196

[174] Bombardier C, Laine L, Reicin A, Shapiro D, Burgos-Vargas R, Davis B et al., Comparison of upper gastrointestinal toxicity of rofecoxib and naproxen in patients with rheumatoid arthritis. N Engl J Med 2000; 343: 1520 – 1528

[175] Catella-Lawson F, McAdam B, Morrison BW, Kapoor S, Kujibu D, Antes L et al. Effect of specific inhibition of cyclooxygenase-2 on sodium balance of, hemodynamics, and vasoactive eicosanoids. J Pharmacol Exp Ther 1999; 289: 735 – 741

[176] Swan SK, Lasseter CK, Ryan CF, Buechel LJ, Lambrecht LJ, Pinto MB et al. Renal effects of multiple dose rofecoxib, a COX-2 inhibitor, in elderly subjects. J Am Soc Nephrol 1999; 10: 641 A [Abstract]

[177] Swan SK, Rudy W, Lasseter CK, Ryan CF, Buechel LJ, Lambrecht LJ et al. Effects of cyclooxygense inhibition on renal function in elderly persons receiving a low salt diet. A randomised controlled trial. Ann Intern Med 2000; 133: 1 – 9

[178] Kargman S, Charleson S, Cartwrigt M, Franc J, Riendeau D, Mancini J. Characterisation of prostaglandin G/H synthase 1 and 2 in rat, dog, monkey and human gastrointestinal tract. Gastroenterology 1996; 111: 445 – 454

[179] Jackson ML, Wu K, Mahida YR. COX-1 expression in human gastric mucosa infected with Helicobacter pylori: constitutive or induced? Gastroenterology 1998; 114: A160

[180] Mclaughlan J, Seth R, Cole AT, Scott BB, Jenkins D, Hawkey CJ. Increased inducible cyclooxygenase associated with treatment failure in ulcerative colitis. Gastroenterology 1996; 110: A964

[181] Wallace JL. Selective COX-2 inhibitors: is the water becoming muddy? TIPS 1999; 20: 4 – 6

[182] Reuter BK, Asfaha S, Buret S, Sharkey K, Wallace JL. Exacerbation of inflammation-associated colonic injury in rat through inhibition of cyclooxygenase-2. J Clin Invest 1996; 98: 2067 – 2085

[183] Mizuno H, Sakamoto C, Matsuda K, Wada K, Uchida T, Noguchi H et al. Induction of cyclooxygenase-2 in gastric mucosal lesions and its inhibition by specific antagonist delays healing in mice. Gastroenterology 1997; 112: 387 – 397

[184] Schmassmann A, Peskar BM, Stettler C, Netzer P, Stroff T, Flogerzi B et al. Effects of inhibition of prostaglandin endoperoxide-2 in chronic gastrointestinal ulcer models in rats. Br J Pharmacol 1998; 123: 795 – 804

[185] Chan CC, Boyge S, Brideau C, Ford-Hutchinson AM, Gordon R, Guay D, Hill RG, Li CS, Wong E, Penneton M, Prasit P, Roy P, Tagari P, Rodger IW. Pharmacology of a selective cyclooxygenase-2 inhibitor, L-745,337: A novel nonsteroidal anti-inflammatory agent with an ulcerogenic sparing effect in rat and non-human primate stomach. J Pharmacol Exp Ther 1995; 274: 1531 – 1537

[186] Wallace JL, McKnight W, Reuter BK, Vergnolle N. NSAID-induced gastric damage in rats: requirement for inhibition of both cyclooxygenase-1 and – 2. Gastroenterology 2000; 119: 706 – 714

[187] Zimmermann KC, Sarbia M, Schör K, Weber AA. Constitutive cyclooxygenase-2 expression in healthy human and rabbit gastric mucosa. Mol Pharmacol 1998; 54: 536 – 540

[188] Velo GP et al. Distribution of prostaglandins in inflammatory exudate. J Path 1973; 111: 149 – 158

[189] Capasso F et al. Pharmacological mediators of various immunological and non-immunological inflammatory reactions produced in the pleural cavity. Agents Actions 1975; 5: 528 – 533

[190] Willoughby DA. Effects of prostaglandins $PGF_{2\alpha}$ and PGE_1 on vascular permeability. J Path Bacteriol 1968; 96: 381 – 387

[191] Willoughby DA. The Heberden Oration, 1974. Human arthritis aplayed to animals models. Towards a better therapy. Ann Rheum Dis 1975; 34: 471 – 478

[192] Willoughby DA, Moore AR, Colville-Nash PR. COX-1, COX-2, and COX-3 and the future treatment of chronic inflammatory disease. Lancet 2000; 355: 646 – 648

[193] Gilroy DW et al. Inducible cyclooxygenase may have anti-inflammatory properties. Nature Med 1999; 5: 698 – 701

[194] Gilroy DW et al. Differential effects of inhibition of isoforms of cyclooxygenase (COX-1, COX-2) in chronic inflammation. Inflamm Res 1998; 47: 79 – 85

[195] Wallace JL et al. Limited anti-inflammatory efficacy of cyclo-oxygenase inhibition in carrageenan-air-pouch inflammation. Br J Pharmacol 1999; 126: 1200 – 1204

[196] Van Ryn J, Pairet M. Clinical experience with cyclooxygenase-2 inhibitors. Inflamm Res 1999; 48: 247 – 254

[197] Harris RC, McKanna JA, Akai Y, Jacobson HR, Dubois RN, Breyer MD. Cyclooxygenase-2 is associated with the macula densa of rat kidney and increases

with salt restriction. J Clin Invest 1994; 94: 2504–2510
198 Lim H et al. Multiple female reproductive failures in cyclooxygenase 2-deficient mice. Cell 91: 197–208
199 Crankshaw DJ, Dyal R. Effects of some naturally occurring prostanoids and some cylooxygenase inhibitors on the contraction of the human uterine segment in vivo. Can J Physiol Pharmacol 1994; 72: 870–874
200 Eric G et al. Leukotrienes, Lipoxins and Hydroxyeicosatetraenoic acids. Methods Mol Biol 1999; 120: 213–247
201 Dixon RA, Diehl RE, Opas E, Rands E, Vickers PJ, Evans JF, Gillard JW, Miller DK. Requirement of a 5-lipoxygenase-activating protein for leukotriene synthesis. Nature 1990; 343: 282–284
202 Denzlinger C. Biology and pathophysiology of leukotrienes. Crit Rev Oncol Hematol 1996; 23: 167–223
203 Ford-Hutchinson AW, Gresser M, Young RN. 5-lipoxygenase. Ann Rev Biochem 1994; 63: 383–417
204 Ford-Hutchinson AW. Regulation of leukotriene biosynthesis. Cancer Metastasis Rev 1994; 13: 257–267
205 Radmark OP. The molecular biology and regulation of 5-lipoxygenase. Respir Crit Care Med 2000; 161: S11–S15
206 Levy BD, Romano M, Chapman HA, Reilly JJ, Drazen J, Serhan CN. Human alveolar macrophages have 15-lipoxygenase and generate 15(S)-hydroxy-5, 8,11-cis-13-trans-eicosatetraenoic acid and lipoxins. J Clin Invest 1993; 92: 1572–1576
207 Nassar GM, Morrow JD, Roberts LJ, Lakkis FG, Badr KF. Induction of 15-lipoxygenase by interleukin-13 in human blood monocytes. J Biol Chem 1994; 269: 27,631
208 Sigal E, Conrad DJ. Human 15-lipoxygenase: a potential effector molecule for interleukin-4. Adv Prostaglandin Thromboxane Leukot Res 1994; 22: 309
209 Katoh T, Lakkis FG, Makita N, Badr KF. Co-regulated expression of glomerular 12/15-lipoxygenase and interleukin-4 mRNA in rat nephrotoxic nephritis. Kidney Int 1994; 46: 341
210 Badr KF, Lakkis FG. Lipoxygenase products in normal and diseased glomeruli. Ann N Y Acad Sci 1994; 744: 216–219
211 Crooke S et al. Leukotriene receptors and signal transduction. Biochem Actions Horm 1987; 14: 81–139
212 Yokomizo T, Izumi T, Chang K, Takuwa Y, Shimizu T. G-protein-coupled receptor for leukotriene B_4 that mediates chemotaxis. Nature 1997; 387: 620–624
213 Yokomizo T, Masude K, Kato K, Toda A, Izumi T, Shimizu T. Leukotriene B receptor: cloning and intracellular signaling. Am J Respir Crit Care Med 2000; 161: S46–S50
214 Drazen JM, Elliot I, O'Bryen PM. Drug therapy: treatment of asthma with drugs modifying the leukotriene pathway. New Engl J Med 1999; 640: 197–206
215 Sarau H et al. Identification and characterisation of leukotriene D_4 receptors and signal transduction processes in rat basophilic leukaemia cells. J Biol Chem 1987; 262: 4034–4041
216 Mong S et al. SKF 104,353, a high affinity antagonist for human and guinea pig lung leukotriene D_4 receptor blocked phosphatidylinositol metabolism and thromboxane synthesis induced by leukotriene D_4. Mol Pharmacol 1987; 32: 223–229
217 Sala A, Testa G, Folco G. Leukotriene A_4 and not Leukotriene B_4 is the main 5-lipoxygenase metabolite released by bovine leukocytes. FEBS Letters 1996; 388: 94–98
218 Sala A, Bolla M, Zarini S, Muller-Peddinghaus R, Folco G. Release of Leukotriene A_4 versus B_4 from human polymorphonuclear leukocytes. J Biol Chem 1986; 271: 17,944–17,948
219 Feinmark SJ, Cannon PJ. Endothelial cell leukotriene C_4 synthesis results from intercellular transfer of leukotriene A_4 synthesised by polymorphonuclear leukocytes. J Biol Chem 1986; 343: 282–284
220 Edenius C, Heidvall K, Lindgren JA. Novel transcellular interaction: conversion of granulocyte-derived leukotriene A_4 to cysteinyl-containing leukotrienes by human platelets. Eur J Biochem 1988; 178: 81–86
221 Brady HR, Papayianni A, Serhan CN. Leukocyte adhesion promotes biosynthesis of lipoxygenase products by transcellular route. Kidney Int 1994; 45: S90–S97
222 Scoggan KA, Ford-Hutchinson AW, Nicholson DW. Differential activation of leukotriene biosynthesis by granulocyte-macrophage colony stimulating factor and interleukin-5 in an eosinophilic substring of HL-60 cells. Blood 1995; 86: 3507–3516
223 Wendy HE, Pelletier JP, Pelletier MJ, Laufer S, Di Battista JA. Synthesis of interleukin 1β, tumor necrosis factor-α, and interstitial collagenase (MMP-1). Is eicosanoid dependent in human osteoarthritis synovial membrane explants: Interactions with anti-inflammatory cytokines. J Rheumatol 2002; 29: 546–553
224 Riddick CA, Serio KJ, Hodulik CR, Ring WL, Regn MS, Bigby TD. TGF-β increases leukotriene C_4 synthase expression in the monocyte-like cell line, THP-1. J Immunol 1999; 162: 1101–1107
225 Brahn E. Animal models of rheumatoid arthritis. Clues to aetiology and treatment. Clin Orth Rel Res 1991; 265: 42–53
226 Ferreira SH, Vane JR. Mode of action of anti-inflammatory agents which are prostaglandin synthesase inhibitors. In: Vane JR, Ferreira SH (eds). Anti-Inflammatory Drugs. Berlin: Springer, 1979: 348–398
227 Heller A, Koch T, Schmeck J, Van Ackern K. Lipid mediators in inflammatory disorders. Drugs 1998; 55: 487–496

[228] Gök S, Ülker S, Hüseyinov A, Hatip FB, Çinar MG, Evinç A. Role of leukotrienes on coronary vasoconstriction in isolated hearts of arthritic rats: effect of in vivo treatment with CI-986, a dual inhibitor of cyclooxygenase and lipoxygenase. Pharmacology 2000; 60: 41 – 46

[229] Shatron P, Stenson WF. Enhanced synthesis of leukotrienes B_4 by colonic mucosa in inflammatory bowel disease. Gastroenterology 1984; 86: 453 – 460

[230] Peskar BM et al. Enhanced formation of sulfidopeptide-leukotrienes in ulcerative colitis and Crohn's disease: inhibitory sulphasalazine and 5-aminosalycilic acid. Agents Actions 1986; 18: 381 – 383

[231] Lewis RA, Austen R. The biologically active leukotrienes. J Clin Invest 1984; 73: 889 – 897

[232] Rahman MA, Nakazawa M, Emancipator SN, Dunn MJ. Increased leukotriene B_4 synthesis in immune injured rat glomeruli. J Clin Invest 1988; 81: 1945 – 1952

[233] Lianos EA. Synthesis of hydroxyeicosatetraenoic acids and leukotrienes in rat nephrotoxic serum nephritis. J Cline Invest 1988; 82: 427 – 435

[234] Creticos PS et al. Peptide leukotrienes release after antigen challenge in patients sensitive to ragweed. New Engl J Med 1984; 310: 1626 – 1630

[235] Naclerio RM et al. Inflammatory mediators in late antigen-induced rhinitis. New Engl J Med 1985; 313: 65 – 70

[236] McMillan RM, Walker ER. Designing therapeutically effective 5-lipoxygenase inhibitors. TIPS 1992; 13: 323 – 330

[237] Rainsford KD. The effects of 5-lipoxygenase inhibitors and leukotriene antagonists on the development of gastric lesions induced by nonsteroidal anti-inflammatory drugs in mice. Agent Actions 1987; 21: 16 – 319

[238] Rainsford KD. Leukotrienes in the pathogenesis of NSAID-induced gastric and intestinal mucosal damage. Agent Actions 1993; 39: C24 – C26

[239] Wallace JL, McKnight GW, Keenan CM, Byles NI, MacNaughton WK. Effects of leukotrienes on susceptibility of the rat stomach to damage and investigation of the mechanism of action. Gastroenterology 1990; 35: 662 – 669

[240] Badr KF, Schreiner GF, Wasserman M, Ichikawa I. Preservation of the glomerular ultrafiltration coefficient during rat nephrotoxic serum nephritis by a specific leukotriene D4 receptor antagonist. J Clin Invest 1988; 81: 1702 – 1709

[241] Katoh T, Lianos EA, Fukunaga M, Takahashi K, Badr KF. Leukotriene D_4 is a mediator of proteinuria and glomerular hemodynamic abnormalities in passive Heymann nephritis. J Clin Invest 1993; 91: 1507 – 1515

[242] Butterly DW, Spurney RF, Ruiz P, Griffiths R, Albrightson C, Coffman T. A role for leukotrienes in cyclosporine nephrotoxicity. Kidney Int 2000; 57: 2586 – 2593

[243] Steinhilber D. 5-Lipoxygenase: a target for anti-inflammatory drugs revisited. Cur Med Chem 1999; 6: 71 – 85

[244] Bruneau P, Delvare C, Edwards MP, McMillan RM. Indazolinones, a new series of redox-active 5-lipoxygenase inhibitors with built-in selectivity and oral activity. J Med Chem 1991; 34: 1028 – 1036

[245] Carter GW, Young PR, Albert DH, Bouska J, Dyer R, Bell RL, Summers JB, Brooks DW. 5-lipoxygenase inhibitory activity of zileuton. J Pharm Exp Ther 1991; 256: 929 – 937

[246] Jackson WP, Islip PJ, Kneen G, Pugh A, Wates PJ. Acetohydroxamic acids as potent, selective, orally active 5-lipoxygenase inhibitors. J Med Chem 1988; 31: 500 – 503

[247] Knapp HR. Reduced allergen-induced nasal congestion and leukotriene synthesis with orally active 5-lipoxygenase inhibitor. New Engl J Med 1990; 323: 1745 – 1748

[248] Weinblatt ME, Kremer JM, Coblyn JS, Helfgott S, Maier AL, Petrillo G, Henson B, Rubin P, Sperling R. Zileuton, a 5-lipoxygenase inhibitor, in rheumatoid arthritis. J Rheumatol 1992; 19: 1537 – 1541

[249] Collawn C, Rubin P, Perez N, Bobadilla J, Cabrera G Reyes E, Borovoy J, Kershenobich D. Phase II study of the safety and efficacy of a 5-lipoxygenase inhibitory in patients with ulcerative colitis. Am J Gastroenterol 1992; 87: 342 – 346

[250] Hawkey CJ, Dube LM, Rountree LV, Linnen PJ, Lancaster JF. A trial of zileuton versus mesalazine or placebo in the maintenance of remission of ulcerative colitis. Gastroenterology 1997; 112: 718 – 724

[251] Bird TGC et al. Methoxyalkyl thiazoles: a new series of potent, selective, and orally active 5-lipoxygenase inhibitors displaying high enantioselectivity. J Med Chem 1991; 34: 2176 – 2186

[252] McMillan RM et al. Methoxyalkyl thiazoles: a novel series of potent, orally active and enantioselective inhibitors of 5-lipoxygenase. Agents Actions 1991; 34: 110 – 112

[253] Kreft AF et al. Conversion of a cyclooxygenase (CO) inhibitor into a 5-lipoxygenase (LO) inhibitor: a general route to novel orally active anti-inflammatory and anti-allergy drugs. Drugs Under Exp Clin Resn 1991; 17: 381 – 387

[254] Guasch A, Zayas CF, Badr KF. MK-591 acutely restores glomerular size selectivity and reduces proteinuria in human glomerulonephritis. Kidney Int 1999; 56: 261 – 267

[255] Roberts WG et al. Leukotrienes in ulcerative colitis: results of a multicenter trial of a leukotriene biosynthesis inhibitor MK-591. Gastroenterology 1997; 112: 725 – 732

[256] Serhan CN. Lipoxins and novel aspirin-triggered 15-epi-lipoxins (ATL): a jungle of cell-cell interactions or a therapeutic opportunity? Prostaglandins 1997; 53: 107 – 137

[257] Claria J, Lee MH, Serhan CN. Aspirin-triggered lipoxins (15-epi-LX) are generated by the human lung adenocarcinoma cell line (A549)-neutrophil

interactions and are potent inhibitors of cell proliferation. Mol Med 1996; 2: 583 – 587

[258] Fiore S, Serhan CN. Formation of lipoxins and leukotrienes during receptor-mediated interactions of human platelets and recombinant human granulocyte/macrophage colony-stimulating factor-primed neutrophils. J Exp Med 1990; 172: 1451 – 1455

[259] Lindgren JA, Edenius C. Transcellular biosynthesis of leukotrienes and lipoxins via leukotriene A_4 transfer. Trends Pharmacol Sci 1993; 14: 351 – 355

[260] Sheppard KA et al. Lipoxin generation by human megakaryocyte-induced 12-lipoxygenase. Biochem Biophys Acta 1992; 1133: 223

[261] Romano M, Serhan CN. Lipoxin generation by permeabilized human platelets. Biochemistry 1992; 31: 8269

[262] Romano M et al. Lipoxin synthase activity of human platelets 12-lipoxygenase. Biochem J 1993; 296: 127

[263] Lehr H-A et al. P-selectin mediates the interaction of circulating leukocytes with platelets and microvascular endothelium in response to oxidized lipoprotein in vivo. Lan Invest 1994; 71: 380

[264] Lehr H-A, Frei B, Arfors K-E. Vitamin C prevents cigarette smoke-induced leukocyte aggregation and adhesion to endothelium in vivo. Proc Natl Acad Sci USA. 1994; 91: 7688

[265] Claria J, Lee MH, Serhan CN. Aspirin-triggered lipoxins (15-epi-LX) are generated by human lung adenocarcinoma cell line (A549)-neutrophil interactions and are potent inhibitors of cell proliferation. Mol Med 1996; 2: 583

[266] Claria J, Serhan CN. Aspirin triggers previously undescribed bioactive eicosanoids by human endothelial cell-leukocyte interactions. Proc Natl Acad Sci USA 1995; 92: 9475 – 9479

[267] Herschman HR. Prostaglandin synthase 2. Biochim Biophys Acta 1996; 1299: 125

[268] Hla T, Nielson K. Human cyclooxygenase-2 cDNA. Proc Natl Acad Sci USA 1992; 89: 7384

[269] Holtzman MJ et al. Prostaglandin H synthase and lipoxygenase gene families in the epithelial cell barrier. Ann N Y Acad Sci 1994; 744: 58

[270] Serhan CN. Lipoxins and novel Aspirin-triggered 15-epi-lipoxins (ATL): A jungle of cell-cell interactions or a therapeutic opportunity? Prostaglandins 1997; 53: 1707 – 1137

[271] Brezinsky ME, Gimbrone MA, Nicolaou KC, Serhan CN. Lipoxins stimulates prostacyclin generation by human endothelial cells. FEBS Lett 1989; 263: 167

[272] Dahlen SE, Franzen L, Raud J et al. Action of lipoxin A_4 and related compounds in smooth muscle preparations and on microcirculation in vivo. Adv Exp Med Biol 1988; 229: 107

[273] Rainsford KD. The effects of 5-lipoxygenase inhibitors and leukotriene antagonists on the development of gastric lesions induced by nonsteroidal anti-inflammatory drugs in mice. Agent and Actions 1987; 21: 16 – 319

[274] Rainsford KD. Leukotrienes in the pathogenesis of NSAID-induced gastric and intestinal mucosal damage. Agent Actions 1993; 39: C24-C26. Gastroenterology 1997; 112: 725 – 732

[275] Hay DWP, Torphy TJ, Unden BJ. Cysteinyl leukotrienes in asthma: old mediators up to new tricks. TIPS 1995; 16: 304 – 309

[276] Raud J, Dahlen SE, Sydbom A, Lindbom L, Hedqvist P. Prostaglandin modulation of mast cell-dependent inflammation. Agents Actions 1989; 26: 42 – 44

[277] Hedqvist P, Raud J, Palmertz U, Kumlin M, Dahlen SE. Eicosanoids as mediators and modulators of inflammation. Adv Prost Thromb Leuk Res 1991; 21 B: 537 – 543

[278] Argentieri DC, Anderson DW, Ritchie DM, Rosenthale ME, Capetola RJ. Tepoxalin inhibits prostaglandin and leukotriene production in adjuvant arthritic rats and in dog knee joints challenged with sodium-urate and immune complex. The FASEB J 1990; 4: 4974

[279] Wallace JL et al. Tissue-selective inhibition of prostaglandin synthesis in rat by tepoxalin: anti-inflammatory without gastropathy. Gastroenterology 1993; 105: 1630 – 1636

[280] Knight EV. Preclinical toxicity evaluation of tepoxalin, a dual inhibitor of cyclooxygenase and 5-lipoxygenase in Sprague Dawley rats and beagle dogs. Fundam Appl Toxicol 1996; 33: 38 – 48

[281] Loomans ME, Matthews RS, Miller J. Novel anti-inflammatory agents. Pharmaceutical compositions and methods for reducing inflammation. US Patent 1987; 4: 708 – 966

[282] Janusz JM et al. New cyclooxygenase-2/5-lipoxygenase inhibitors. 1. 7-tert-buty1 – 2, 3-dihydro-3, 3-dimethylbenzofuran derivatives as gastrointestinal safe anti-inflammatory and analgesic agents: discovery and variation of the 5-keto substituent. J Med Chem 1998; 41: 1112 – 1123

[283] Weisman SM, Doyle MJ, Weheyer KR, Hynd BA, Eichold TH. Effect of tebufelone (NE-11,740), a new anti-inflammatory drug, on arachidonic acid metabolism. Agents Actions 1994; 41: 256 – 263

[284] Powell JH, Meredith MP, Vargas R, McMahon FG, Jain AK. Antipyretic activity of tebufelone (NE-11,740) in man. Agents Actions 1991; 32: 45 – 49

[285] Guttendorf RJ, Andress LD, Shailer P. Single-dose pharmacokinetics and dose proportionality of the anti-inflammatory drug, CI-1004, in healthy subjects. Pharmac Res 1997; 14: A818

[286] Guttendorf RJ, Andress LD, Shailer P. Multiple-dose pharmacokinetics of the anti-inflammatory drug, CI-1004, in healthy subjects after 3-weeks of once-daily dosing. Pharmac Res 1997; 14: A818

[287] Wong S, Lee SJ, Frierson III MR, Proch J, Miskowski TA, Rigby BS, Schomlka SJ, Naismith RW, Kreutzer DC, Lindquist R. Antiarthritic profile of BF-389, a novel anti-inflammatory agent with low ulcerogenic liability. Agents Actions 1992; 37: 90 – 98

[288] Malloy EA, Beers SA, Wachter M. RWJ 63,556, a potent orally active dual 5-LO/COX-2 inhibitor: in vi-

tro and in vivo pharmacology. 24th American Chemical Society National Meeting 1997; A 091

289 Kirchner T, Argentieri DC, Barbone AG, Singer M, Steber M, Ansell J, Beers SA, Wachter MP, Wu W, Malloy E, Stewart A, Ritchie DM. Evaluation of the anti-inflammatory activity of a dual cyclooxygenase-2 selective/5-lipoxygenase inhibitor, RWJ 63,556, in a canine model of inflammation. J Pharmacol Exp Ther 1997; 282: 1094–1101

290 Knight PM, Scherz MW, Cruze CA, Wehmeyer KR. Analysis of a novel anti-inflammatory agent, 1-(7-tert.-butyl-2,3-dihydro-3, 3-dimethylbenzo(b)furan-5-yl)-4- cyclopylbutan-1-one (PGV-20,229), in plasma matrices by stable-isotope-dilution gas chromatography-mass spectrometry. J Chrom 1997; 700: 111

291 Laufer S, Tries S, Augustin J, Elsasser R, Algate DR, Atterson PR, Munt PL. Gastrointestinal tolerance of [2,2-dimethyl-6-(4-chlorophenyl-7-phenyl-2, 3-dihydro-1 H–pyrrolizine-5-yl]-acetic acid in the rat. Arnz-Forsch/Drug Res 1994; 44: 1329–1333

292 Wallace JL, Carter L, McKnight W, Tries S, Laufer S. ML 3000 reduces gastric prostaglandin synthesis without causing mucosal injury. Eur J Pharmacol 1994; 271: 525–531

293 Tries S, Laufer S. The pharmacological profile of ML3000: A new pyrrolizine derivate inhibiting the enzymes cyclo-oxygenase and 5-lipoxygenase. Inflammopharmacology 2001; 9: 113–124

294 Chin B, Wallace J. ML3000. Current Opinion in CPNS Investigational Drugs 1999; 1: 148–152

295 Wallace JL et al. ML3000 reduces gastric prostaglandin synthesis without causing mucosal injury. Europ J of Pharmacol 1994; 271: 525–531

296 Laufer S. Discovery and development of ML3000. Inflammopharmacology 2001; 9: 101–112

297 Algate DR, Agustin J, Atterson PR, Beard DJ, Jobling CM, Laufer S, Munt PL, Tries S. General pharmacology of (2,2-Dimethyl-6- (4-chlorophenyl)-7-phenyl-2, 3-dihydro-1 H–pyrrolizine)-acetic acid in experimental animals. Arzneimittelforschung 1995; 45: 159–165

298 Laufer S, Tries S, Augustin J, Dannhardt G. Pharmacological profile of a new pyrrolozine derivative inhibiting the enzymes cyclooxygenase and 5-lipoxygenase. Arzneim-Forsch/Drug Res 1994; 44: 629–636

299 Laufer S, Tries S, Augustin J, Elsasser R, Albrecht W, Guserle R, Algate DR, Atterson PR, Munt PL. Acute and chronic anti-inflammatory properties of (2,2-dimethyl-6-(4-chlorophenyl)-7-phenyl-2, 3-dihydro-1H-pyrrolizine-5-yl)-acetic acid. Arsenic-Frost/Drug Res 1995; 45: 27–23

300 Laufer SA, Augustin J, Dannhardt G, Kiefer W. 6,7-Diaryldihydropyrrolizin-5-yl)acetic acids, a novel class of potent dual inhibitors of both cyclooxygenase and 5-lipoxygenase. J Med Chem 1994; 37: 1894–1897

301 Gay RE, Neidhart M, Pataky F, Tries S, Laufer S, Gay S. Dual inhibition of 5-lipoxygenase and cyclooxygenases-1 and -2 by ML 3000 reduces joint destruction in adjuvant arthritis. J Rheumatol 2001; 28: 2060–2065

302 Jovanovic DV, Fernandes JC, Martel-Pelletier J, Jolicoeur FC, Reboul P, Laufer S, Tries S, Pelletier JP. In vivo dual inhibition of cyclooxygenase and lipoxygenase by ML-3000 reduces the progression of experimental osteoarthritis: suppression of collagenase 1 and interleukin-1 beta synthesis. Arthritis Rheum 2001; 44: 2320–2330

303 Deigner HP, Freyberg CE, Laufer S. Distribution and excretion of [14 C]-labelled [2,2-dimethyl-6-(4-chlorophenyl)-7-phenyl-2, 3-dihydro-1H-pyrrolizine-5-yl]-[2′-14 C]-acetic acid in rats. Arzneim-Forsch/Drug Res 1995; 45: 272–276

304 Tries S, Neupert W, Laufer S. The mechanism of action of the new anti-inflammatory compound ML 3000: inhibition of 5-LOX and COX-1/2. Inflamm Res 2002; 51: 135–143

305 Hudson N, Balsitis M, Everitt S, Hawkey CJ. Enhanced gastric mucosal leukotriene B_4 synthesis in patients taking non-steroidal anti-inflammatory drugs. Gut 1993; 34: 742–747

306 Pihan G, Rogers C, Szabo S. Vascular injury in acute gastric mucosal damage. Mediatory role of leukotrienes. Dig Dis Sci 1988; 33: 625–632

307 Kobayashi K, Fukuda T, Higuchi K, Nakamura H, Arakawa T. Role of leukotrienes in indomethacin-induced mucosal damage in rats. J Clin Gastroenterol 1993; 17 (Suppl 1): S11–4

308 Rotondo S, Dell'Elba G, Manarini S, Martelli N, Simone V, Evangelista V, Cerletti C. ML 3000, a balanced inhibitor of cyclooxygenase and lipoxygenase, inhibits platelet/polymorphonuclear leukocytes metabolism and adhesion. BR J Pharmacol 2001; 133 (Suppl)

309 Tries S, Laufer S, Radziwon P, Breddin K. Antithrombotic and platelet function inhibiting effects of ML3000, a new anti-inflammatory drug with COX/5-LOX inhibitory activity. Inflamm Res 2002; 51: 129–134

310 Fiorucci S, Distrutti E, Mencarelli A, Palazzetti B, Morelli A. A Dual cyclo-and lipo-oxygenase inhibition, ML3000 spares the gastric mucosa in aspirin treated rats. Gut 2001; 49 (Suppl 3)

311 Jovanovic DV et al. In vivo dual inhibition of cyclooxygenase and lipoxygenase by ML-3000 reduces the progression of experimental osteoarthritis: suppression of collagenase 1 and interleukin-1 beta syhthesis. Arthritis Rheum 2001; 44: 2320–2330

312 Christelle B et al. Licofelone (ML-3000), a dual inhibitor of 5-lipoxygenase and cyclooxygenase, reduces the level of cartilage chondrocyte death *in vivo* in experimental dog osteoarthritis: inhibition of pro-apoptotic factor S. 2002; in press

3 Drug Therapy Today

Kay Brune

A wide range of drugs are currently available for the treatment of rheumatic diseases. The spectrum of activity of some of them is rather narrow, being limited almost solely to analgesia (acetaminophen, opioids) or anti-inflammatory action (glucocorticoids). By contrast, the nonsteroidal anti-inflammatory drugs (NSAIDs) have both analgesic and anti-inflammatory properties. Finally, the disease-modifying antirheumatic drugs (DMARDs), also referred to as slow-acting antirheumatic drugs (SAARDs), have a very complex mode of action that often includes an immunomodulating, immunosuppressive, or cytostatic component.

Inflammatory rheumatic diseases are usually treated with NSAIDs. Analgesics without anti-inflammatory activity are rarely used alone in this indication but almost exclusively to support treatment.

By contrast, acetaminophen (paracetamol) with its analgesic and antipyretic action was, until recently, the drug of first choice for the treatment of painful arthritis. Today the cyclooxygenase-2 (COX-2)-selective inhibitors are being used to an increasing extent.

In chronic (rheumatoid) arthritis DMARDs are used in addition to NSAIDs and glucocorticoids. If they too prove ineffective, so-called biologicals can be used.

This chapter focuses on the established analgesics and anti-inflammatory drugs that have been widely used for some time in the treatment rheumatic disease. It also deals extensively with the modern COX-2 inhibitors. Therapeutic approaches with which little or no clinical experience has so far been gained are the subject of the next chapter.

3.1 Nonsteroidal anti-inflammatory drugs

Thanks to their analgesic, antipyretic, and anti-inflammatory action, the nonsteroidal anti-inflammatory drugs (NSAIDs) are the drugs of first choice for the treatment of most painful rheumatic diseases. They are used in acute arthritis (including gout attacks), chronic arthritis (particularly rheumatoid arthritis), ankylosing spondylitis and other inflammatory diseases of the spine, acute inflammation associated with degenerative diseases of the joints and spine, and acute pain syndromes associated with rheumatic diseases of soft tissues.

Mechanism of action

NSAIDs act essentially by inhibiting the synthesis of prostaglandins and thromboxanes, a group of lipid mediators formed from arachidonic acid. Arachidonic acid is released by phospholipase A_2 from cell-membrane phospholipids and is converted by prostaglandin-H_2-(PGH_2) synthase to prostaglandins. PGH_2 synthase is a membrane-bound enzyme that occurs ubiquitously in the human body. Often for the sake of simplicity PGH_2 synthase is equated with cyclooxygenase. Strictly speaking, however, it is a bifunctional enzyme combining the activity of a cyclooxygenase (COX) and that of a hydroperoxidase (HOX). Thus, in the first enzymatic step prostaglandin G_2 is formed, which is then immediately converted to prostaglandin H_2. The most important inflammatory mediator formed from arachidonic acid via the COX metabolic pathway is prostaglandin E_2 (PGE_2). A second enzyme, 5-lipoxygenase, converts arachidonic acid to leukotrienes and HPETEs (hydroperoxyeicosatetraenoic acids (Fig. 3.**1**).

PGE_2 is a potent dilator of smooth vascular muscle and, as a result of this action, is responsible for the characteristic reddening and vasodilation associated with acute inflammatory processes. Although PGE_2 does not in itself cause pain, it potentiates the activity of other mediators involved in the development of inflammatory pain by sensitizing afferent nerve endings to the effects of bradykinin and histamine [Ferreira, 1972]. Moreover, PGE_2 is released in the CNS, producing fever [Saxena et al., 1979].

In addition to PGE_2, numerous other substances formed by COX have been identified in inflamed tissues, e.g. $PGF_{2\alpha}$, PGD_2, prostacyclin (PGI_2) and thromboxane A_2 (TXA_2). Of these, prostacyclin is probably the most significant in the context of inflammation, as it also has a marked vasodilating effect, and its pain-intensifying action is even more pronounced than that of PGE_2. Prostaglandins, thromboxanes, and leukotrienes are collectively referred to as eicosanoids, as they can all be derived from the hypothetical fatty acid prostanoic acid which contains 20 (Greek *eikosi*) carbon atoms. Prostaglandins and thromboxanes are also subsumed under the term prostanoids. Because of their rapid metabolic inactivation, the prostanoids are only active for a few seconds to minutes at the site of their synthesis and therefore have to be continuously replenished.

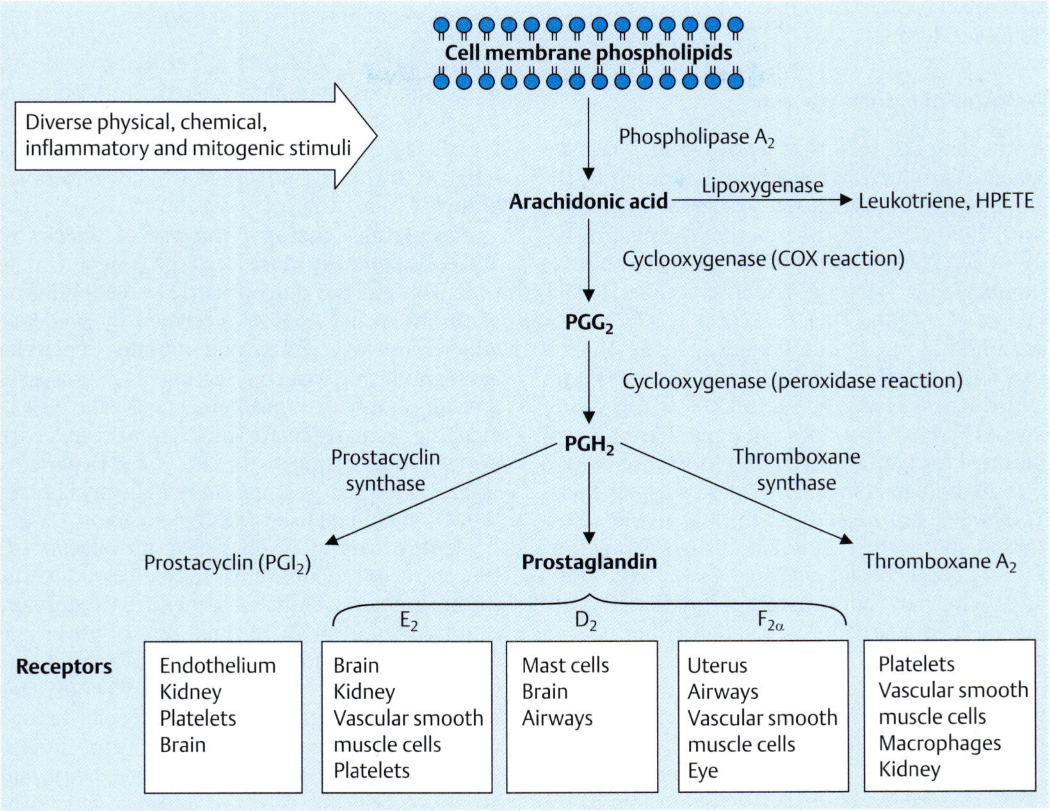

Fig. 3.**1** Prostaglandin, thromboxane and leukotriene: development from arachidonic acid and tissue-specific effects (modified from FitzGerald and Patrono, 2001).

The eicosanoids formed by the body under physiologic conditions carry out a number of functions that can essentially be described as organ-protective or cytoprotective. Thus, prostaglandins are involved in maintaining normal functioning of the gastrointestinal mucosa and kidneys, while thromboxane A_2 has a vasoconstrictive action and is responsible for platelet aggregation in connection with the blood clotting system. Prostacyclin is the most important prostanoid in terms of glomerular hemodynamics; in this context it evidently acts as an antiplatelet and vasodilatory counterpart to thromboxane A_2.

Unlike acetylsalicylic acid, which is irreversibly inactivated by cyclooxygenase via transacetylation, NSAIDs such as indomethacin and ibuprofen are competitive COX inhibitors that compete for the binding site on the enzyme with the substrate arachidonic acid.

The clinical effects of NSAIDs can be adequately explained in terms of their inhibition of prostaglandin synthesis and their substance-specific properties. The acidic NSAIDs such as diclofenac accumulate primarily in the blood, liver, spleen and bone marrow as well as in tissues with an acidic extracellular pH. The latter include inflamed tissues as well as the wall of the upper gastrointestinal tract and the collecting tubules of the kidneys. In inflamed tissue the acidic NSAIDs prevent the pathologic overproduction of prostaglandins and thus the inflammatory reactions triggered primarily by PGE_2 [Brune and Zeilhofer, 1999].

Neutral analgesics (acetaminophen) and weakly alkaline NSAIDs (phenazone and its derivatives, e.g. dipyrone), by contrast, are distributed rapidly and homogeneously throughout the body and are even able to cross the blood-brain barrier. Hence, they are only weak inhibitors of prostaglandin synthesis in the periphery and do not exhibit the side effects on the gastrointestinal tract, the kidneys, and the blood-clotting system that are typical of the acidic NSAIDs [Brune und Zeilhofer, 1999].

Isoforms of cyclooxygenase

It was long assumed that the amounts of prostaglandins produced were determined solely by the availability of the substrate arachidonic acid. Not until 1990 was it discovered that the neosynthesis of a COX enzyme could be induced in human monocytes by bacterial lipopolysaccharide (LPS) [Fu et al., 1990]. This induction is blocked by dexamethasone. In subsequent investigations it was found that inducible COX is a separate isoenzyme. It was given the name COX-2. This isoenzyme is coded by a different gene than the constitutive form, COX-1. The two forms are around 60% homologous in their amino acid sequences. The two isoenzymes differ in their tissue distribution and in the regulation of their expression. COX-1 occurs continuously in nearly all cell types and carries out "housekeeping" functions by producing prostaglandins for regulating normal cell processes. COX-2 has a shorter life and is produced mainly in stress situations, e.g. in response to tissue damage and inflammation. Thus, enhanced COX-2 activity has been measured in the synovial tissue of patients with rheumatoid arthritis and osteoarthritis [Hinz und Brune, 2002].

In view of these findings, it was proposed that the pharmacologic inhibition of constitutive COX-1 is responsible for the adverse effects, while the inhibition of inducible COX-2 is responsible for the therapeutic effects of NSAIDs. If this hypothesis is correct, it should be possible to avoid the risks associated with the use of conventional NSAIDs, especially the risk of gastrointestinal ulcers, by selectively inhibiting COX-2. Meanwhile several COX-2-specific inhibitors (known as coxibs) have been developed, and extensive clinical experience has already been gained with them (see below).

In the wake of recent findings, the initial euphoria has now given way to the sobering insight that the dichotomous division into "good" and "bad" COX isoenzymes is a gross oversimplification. In fact, COX-2 also appears to carry out a number of physiologic tasks, e.g. in connection with wound and ulcer healing, the regulation of intraocular pressure, renal perfusion, and female reproductive functions (Fig. 3.**2**) [overview in Hinz and Brune, 2002].

Common adverse effects of NSAIDs

Treatment with NSAIDs leads to typical side effects due to the pharmacologic inhibition of physiologic prostaglandin synthesis. Substance-specific adverse effects are discussed in the sections on the individual substances and substance groups.

Antiplatelet therapy. The use of NSAIDs in anti-inflammatory doses can prolong bleeding time. This effect is due primarily to the inhibition of thromboxane A_2 (TXA_2) formed by platelets, which removes an important stimulus of platelet aggregation and vasoconstriction. Both processes are important for rapid hemostasis. The risk of bleeding is particularly high in patients with pre-existing clotting disturbances and in patients receiving anticoagulant therapy; in such cases NSAIDs should be used with great care.

Nephrotoxicity. NSAIDs have no relevant effect on renal function in patients with a healthy cardiovascular system. However, NSAID therapy is associated with slight inhibition of water and electrolyte excretion and slightly increased systolic and diastolic blood pressure. There have been isolated reports of acute renal failure, which, however, was favored by special circumstances. Patients with kidney disease, heart failure, hypertension, shock or volume deficiency, and those on diuretic therapy would appear to be particularly at risk. Evidently, prostaglandins (PGI_2, PGE_2) counteract renal vasoconstriction and sodium and water retention in situations of increased renin, angiotensin, and sympathetic activity so as to maintain renal perfusion [Henrich, 1988]. If patients with the aforementioned risk factors are nevertheless treated with NSAIDs, serum creatinine should be closely monitored. The nephrotoxicity is usually reversible on discontinuation of the NSAID. The concurrent use of diuretics or ACE inhibitors can lead to drug interactions (see below).

Gastrointestinal toxicity. Most NSAIDs are weak organic acids. In the acidic milieu of the gastric juice they therefore occur in the undissociated form, which favors their absorption. In the higher pH within cells they redissociate and consequently do not migrate readily out of the cell again. As a result NSAIDs can reach high concentrations in the gastric mucosa and lead to mucosal erosions and ulcers. COX inhibition exacerbates the lesions, since both the acid-secretion-inhibiting activity of PGE_2 and the mucosal protective effects of PGI_2, PGE_2, and $PGF_{2\alpha}$ are

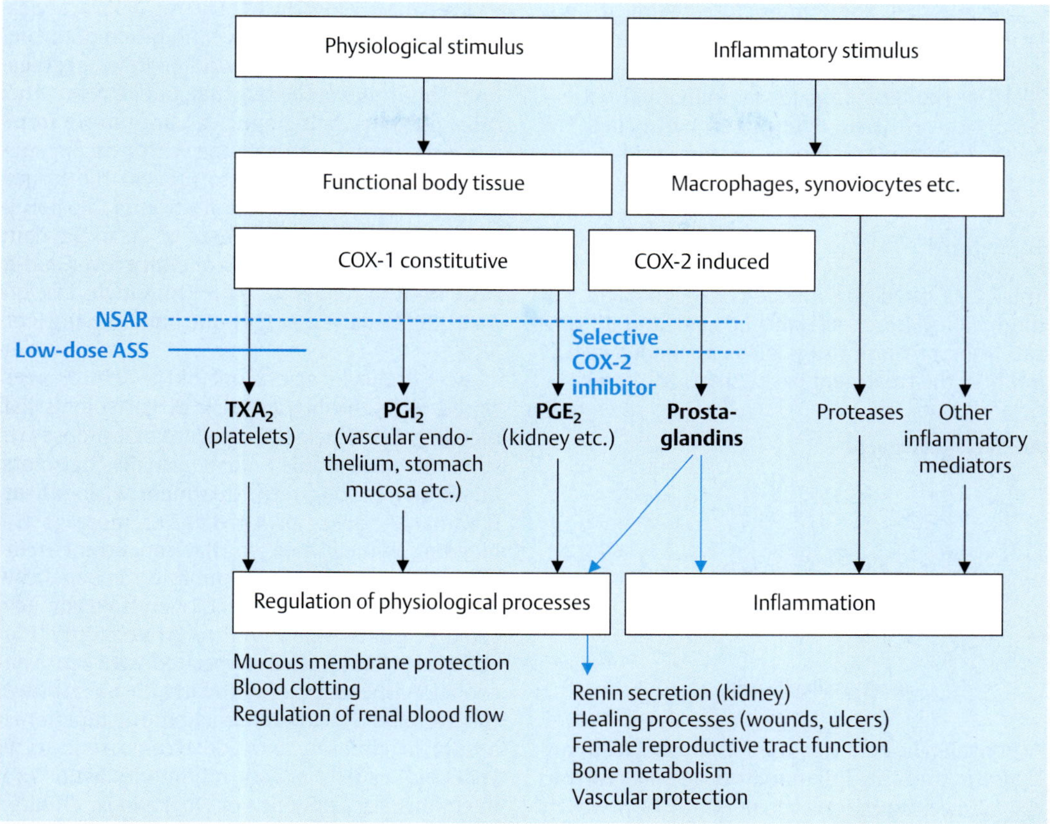

Fig. 3.**2** Physiological and pathophysiological functions of the two isoenzymes COX-1 and COX-2 (modified from Vane and Botting, 1996). ----- reversible inhibition; —— irreversible inhibition

blocked. At least 10–20% of patients on NSAIDs therefore complain of more or less pronounced gastric distress [Wolfe et al., 1999]. 2–4% of patients develop severe complications such as bleeding gastric or duodenal ulcers or perforations. Blood loss is further increased by TXA_2 inhibition and the related prolongation of bleeding time.

Tocolysis. PGE_2 and $PGF_{2\alpha}$ stimulate uterine contractions. NSAIDs can therefore be used for tocolysis. Long-term use of NSAIDs, particularly acetylsalicylic acid, during pregnancy can lead to premature bleeding, prolongation of gestation, delayed onset of labor, birth complications, and, as a result of TXA_2 synthesis inhibition, postpartal bleeding.

Ophthalmic symptoms. The administration of NSAIDs to animals led to adverse effects on the eyes. Therefore, any visual disturbances or ocular changes that occur in a patient on an NSAID should be clarified immediately by an ophthalmologist.

Drug interactions. Most NSAIDs have a high plasma-protein binding rate. They can therefore displace other drugs from their protein binding sites, increase the free plasma concentration of those drugs, and enhance their biological activity or cause toxic effects. Such a risk of drug interactions exists, for example, with coumarin-type anticoagulants, hydantoin, sulfonamides, and sulfonyl ureas. Many NSAIDs are metabolized by hepatic microsomal enzymes. Interactions and substrate competition can therefore occur with drugs that are metabolized by the same enzyme system. Moreover, drugs that act as enzyme inductors can reduce the plasma half-life of NSAIDs. Finally, antacids reduce the bioavailability of NSAIDs, while NSAIDs, in turn, reduce the efficacy of diuretics. Whenever the possibility of a drug interaction exists, the patient needs to be closely monitored.

Despite their sometimes close chemical similarity, there are differences between the pharmacokinetics, efficacy, and tolerability of the NSAIDs. The best drug for an individual patient should therefore be determined by testing. The most important members of the various substance classes are briefly characterized below.

Salicylates

This class of NSAIDs includes salicylic acid, sodium salicylate, acetylsalicylic acid, and diflunisal. None of these drugs plays a significant role today in the treatment of rheumatic diseases.

Acetylsalicylic acid

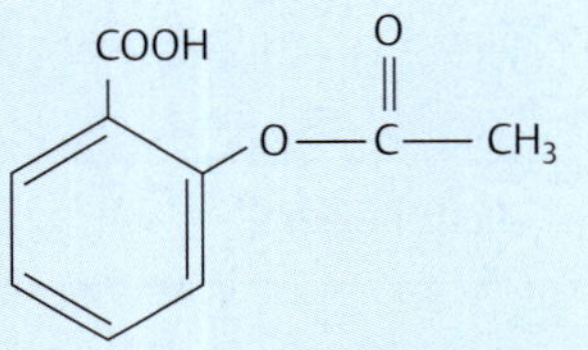

Acetylsalicylic acid

Acetylsalicylic acid was used as an analgesic, antipyretic, and anti-inflammatory agent as early as the 19th century. However, not until 1971 was its mechanism of action as a COX inhibitor elucidated [Vane, 1971] – a pioneering achievement that later earned the discoverer the Nobel Prize. Acetylsalicylic acid acetylates the enzyme and in doing so irreversibly inactivates the catalytic cyclooxygenase center; peroxidase activity remains intact.

The substance undergoes rapid hydrolytic conversion to salicylic acid within 15–30 minutes. Salicylic acid is the actual vehicle of the analgesic and – in higher doses (> 3 g daily) – anti-inflammatory activity. The substance has been detected in numerous tissues, including the synovium. Salicylic acid crosses the blood-brain barrier as well as the placental barrier and is secreted into human breast milk. The elimination rate depends on the dose. Because salicylic acid in high doses is eliminated more slowly than it is absorbed, accumulation of the substance can occur. Depending on the dosage form (effervescent tablet, chewable tablet, coated tablet, delayed-release tablet), salicylic acid reaches peak plasma concentrations after 20 minutes to three hours.

Even in very low doses of 50 mg daily acetylsalicylic acid leads to selective inhibition of thrombocytic TXA_2 production and platelet aggregation. This is due to the fact that, unlike most other cells, platelets, being anuclear, are unable to replace the inactivated enzyme with new enzyme. Therapists use this effect to prevent the formation of coronary and cerebral thrombi in patients with atherosclerosis. In doses of up to 3 g daily acetylsalicylic acid is used to reduce fever and to treat mild to moderate pain. Only high doses of 4–8 g daily have a potent anti-inflammatory effect.

Acetylsalicylic acid is one of the NSAIDs associated with the highest risk of gastrointestinal bleeding. Even the occasional use of low doses results in measurable, albeit usually harmless, blood loss. In long-term treatment with anti-inflammatory doses of 4 g daily or more gastric bleeding is inevitable, so that concurrent treatment with a proton pump inhibitor is beneficial. As a specific adverse effect, acetylsalicylic acid can precipitate Reye's syndrome in children [Pinsky et al., 1988]. This is associated with acute encephalopathy together with fatty degeneration of the liver and disturbed mitochondrial function. It occurs in children and adolescents four to 16 years old, usually in connection with acute viral infections, e.g. influenza or chickenpox. Children should therefore not receive acetylsalicylic acid if possible.

Arylpropionic acid derivatives

Although drugs such as flurbiprofen, ketoprofen, ibuprofen, and naproxen all share a basic arylpropionic acid structure, the molecules differ markedly. All members of this drug class are characterized by good activity in inflammatory processes of the joints and relatively good tolerability.

Ibuprofen

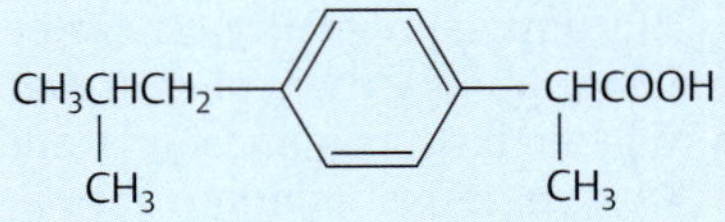

Ibuprofen

In over-the-counter doses of up to 400 mg t.i.d. ibuprofen is mainly effective as an analgesic and antipyretic, less so as an anti-inflammatory drug.

In daily doses of 2.4 g the anti-inflammatory effect of ibuprofen is approximately equivalent to that of 150 mg diclofenac. The total daily dose of ibuprofen should not exceed 2400 mg.

After oral administration ibuprofen is almost fully absorbed, irrespective of simultaneous food intake. Peak plasma levels are reached after about 20 minutes to two hours, depending on the dosage form. Ibuprofen is nearly 100% bound to serum albumin. Because of its short half-life of two hours, ibuprofen can be used "as required" for treating transient pain. In chronic inflammatory conditions ibuprofen must be taken several times daily in order to achieve a constant anti-inflammatory effect. Ibuprofen is almost fully metabolized and eliminated by the kidneys within 24 hours.

Ibuprofen is generally safe and is even tolerated by patients who have encountered gastric problems with acetylsalicylic acid. In high doses, however, ibuprofen can also lead to irritation and bleeding of the gastric mucosa. Furthermore, there have been reports of skin rash, peripheral edema, anorexia, tinnitus, dizziness, and central nervous symptoms such as anxiety, headache, agitation, and visual disturbances. Isolated cases of serious side effects have been reported, e.g. agranulocytosis, aplastic anemia, acute renal failure, interstitial nephritis, and nephrotic syndrome; ibuprofen, after all, is one of the world's most widely used drugs. Ibuprofen can elevate plasma levels of lithium, reduce the renal excretion of methotrexate, and inhibit the natriuretic activity of furosemide.

Naproxen

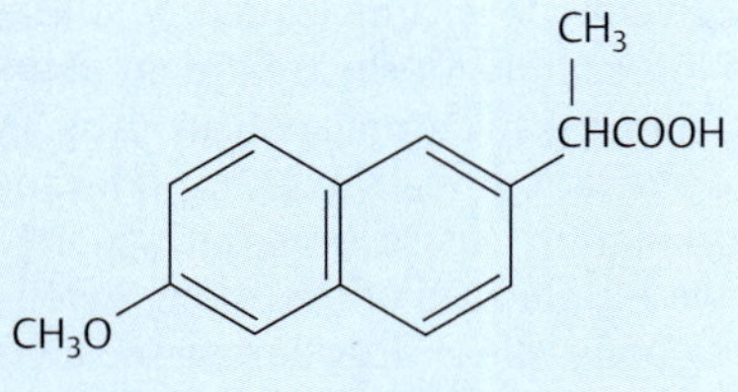

Naproxen

Naproxen, a naphthylpropionic acid derivative, is a well-tolerated NSAID of moderate strength. Following oral administration of the sodium salt it is rapidly and well absorbed, peak plasma levels being reached after one hour. However, its bioavailability is impaired by antacids. Because of its long serum half-life of 13 – 18 hours, naproxen only has to be taken once or twice daily, even for the treatment of chronic inflammatory pain. This can be especially advantageous in patients with compliance problems. In adults a total daily dose of 1500 mg should not be exceeded, though the maximum recommended dose is 750 – 1000 mg daily. Experience with naproxen in pediatric indications has been mainly in the treatment of juvenile chronic arthritis. Typical adverse effects are lethargy and central nervous disturbances.

Arylacetic acid derivatives

This structural class includes diclofenac (aceclofenac), lonazolac, ketorolac, and indomethacin (acemetacin). Aceclofenac and acemetacin are prodrugs. Lonazolac and keterolac play no role in therapeutic practice in Germany. (The same applies to flurbiprofen and ketoprofen, which resemble diclofenac in their pharmacokinetics and indomethacin in their pharmacodynamics.) All these highly effective substances have a short half-life of a few hours and are therefore taken two to three times daily in the treatment of chronic polyarthritis. Here we can only deal in detail with diclofenac and indomethacin.

Diclofenac

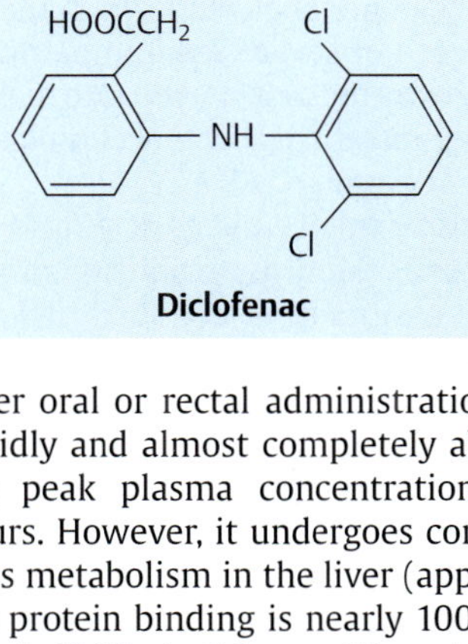

Diclofenac

After oral or rectal administration diclofenac is rapidly and almost completely absorbed, reaching peak plasma concentrations within 2 – 3 hours. However, it undergoes considerable first-pass metabolism in the liver (approx. 50%). Plasma protein binding is nearly 100%, the elimination half-life 1 – 2 hours. Like other NSAIDs with a short half-life, diclofenac accumulates in the synovium and is eliminated significantly more slowly from this compartment than from plasma. Diclofenac is metabolized in the liver, and 90% of the administered substance is excreted in the first 1.5 – 2.5 hours (60% in the urine, 40% in the feces).

Diclofenac is an extremely effective inhibitor of COX, so that gastrointestinal bleeding and ulceration are among the most common side effects. Moderate transaminase elevations have also been observed regularly but were rarely associated with clinical disturbances of hepatic function.

Indomethacin

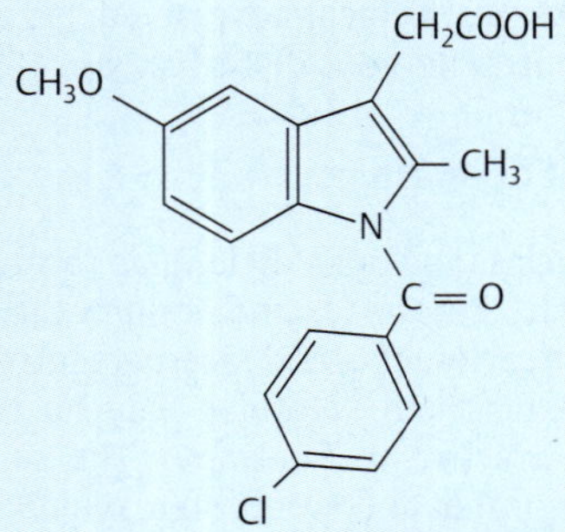

Indomethacin

Indomethacin is also a highly effective NSAID. It is rapidly and completely absorbed from the gastrointestinal tract and is bound almost 100% to plasma proteins. Peak plasma levels are reached after 0.5 to 3 hours. As a result of enterohepatic recirculation, the plasma half-life varies within a broad range (2 – 11 hours). Normally some 30% of the substance is excreted unchanged in the urine and a further 30% in metabolized form in the feces. In the presence of severe renal impairment indomethacin is excreted at a slowed rate mainly via the biliary and intestinal route; accumulation of the substance is possible.

Although it also exhibits analgesic effects, indomethacin is used mainly as an anti-inflammatory drug in the treatment of both arthritis and extra-articular inflammation. The potent inhibition of eicosanoid production inhibits the migration of polymorphonuclear leukocytes into the inflamed area. Thanks to this property indomethacin is an excellent agent for the treatment of acute gout attack. It has also been used successfully to suppress premature labor. If possible indomethacin should not be used in infants and children. However, it has proved effective in closing the patent ductus arteriosus in neonates, since vasodilatory prostaglandins have been implicated in the pathogenesis of this anomaly.

Indomethacin is associated with a relatively high rate of sometimes fatal side effects. Patients therefore need to be informed about the risks and must be carefully monitored. The most common gastrointestinal symptoms are abdominal pain, nausea, vomiting, and gastric and duodenal ulcers. Central nervous side effects include severe frontal headache, dizziness, drowsiness, and depressive and psychotic reactions. In view of this toxicity, use of indomethacin should be limited to short periods.

Thiazinecarboxamides

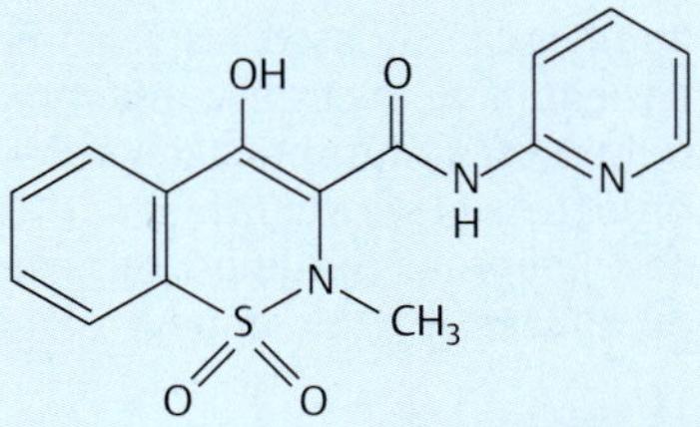

Piroxicam

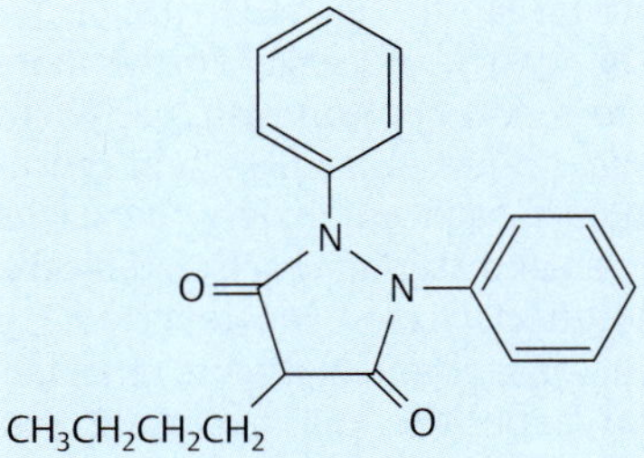

Phenylbutazone

The oxicams **piroxicam** and **tenoxicam** have an extremely long half-life of 40 and 70 hours, respectively. With the usual regimen of 20 mg once daily, constant plasma levels are not reached for several days. Consequently, these drugs are suitable mainly for the treatment of intense chronic pain, e.g. in chronic polyarthritis. In the absence of hepatic impairment, no relevant (further) accumulation occurs, even during long-term use. However, because of their long dwelling time in the body, these drugs are associated with a high rate of gastrointestinal and renal side effects. The elimination half-life of **lornoxicam,** a more recent oxicam, is just four hours so that the substance can be given two or three times daily (8 mg b.i.d. or 4 mg t.i.d.). The short elimination half-life also allows the drug to be used for the treatment of transient pain. The side effects and interactions correspond to those of other NSAIDs but, because of the absence of enterohepatic circulation, ulceration of the lower intestinal segments is rare. In a comparative study of patients with chronic polyarthritis lornoxicam proved equivalent to diclofenac in efficacy.

Phenylbutazone is an effective anti-inflammatory drug with a very slow elimination rate (> 3 days!). Because of its potentially severe side effects (disturbances of hematopoiesis, skin reactions, sodium and water retention with edema, hepatic and renal functional disturbances) phenylbutazone may only be used for short periods after therapeutic alternatives have been exhausted. It is therefore used chiefly in the treatment of gout attacks and acute inflammatory episodes of chronic polyarthritis or Bekhterev's disease.

Selective COX-2 inhibitors (coxibs)

The coxibs, a new group of anti-inflammatory drugs, were developed in response to the unsatisfactory adverse-effect profile of the classical NSAIDs. Both NSAIDs and coxibs inhibit prostaglandin G/H synthase, the enzyme that catalyzes the conversion of arachidonic acid to prostaglandins and thromboxanes. However, whereas the NSAIDs inhibit both known isoforms of the enzyme, COX-1 and COX-2, the coxibs are selective inhibitors of COX-2. They were therefore expected to exhibit significantly better gastrointestinal tolerability. To date two products are commercially available in most countries, celecoxib and rofecoxib. Several others, including etoricoxib, valdecoxib, and the valdecoxib prodrug, parecoxib, which is water-soluble and therefore injectable, are currently undergoing or have recently passed regulatory review.

Celecoxib

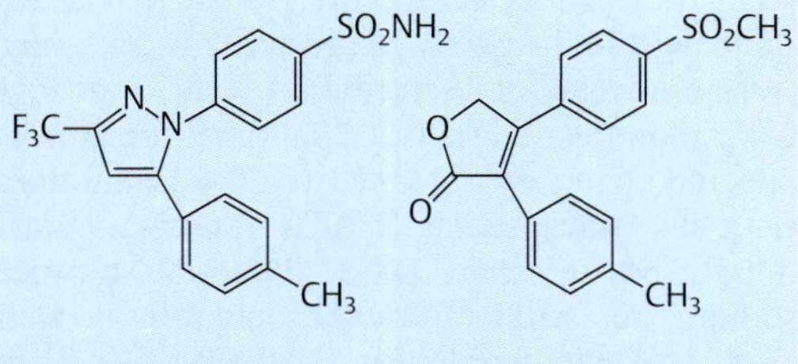

Celecoxib Rofecoxib

Celecoxib was first introduced on the US market in 1999 and has been approved in Germany for the treatment of rheumatoid arthritis and activated osteoarthritis since May 2000. It has a COX-2 specificity, defined as the ratio of the IC_{50} inhibitory concentration for COX-2 and COX-1 in the human whole blood assay, of 7.6 [Riendeau et al., 2001]. Following an oral dose peak, plasma concentrations are reached after 2–3 hours. When celecoxib is taken with a high-fat meal, the time to peak plasma concentration is delayed by about one hour. The drug's oral bioavailability is approximately 60–70%. Over 90% of the substance is bound to plasma proteins. Celecoxib crosses the placental barrier and is secreted into human breast milk. With an elimination half-life of 8–12 hours, steady-state concentrations are reached after two days of treatment. However, much of the pharmacokinetic data on celecoxib are still contradictory and confusing. Celecoxib is metabolized by CYP2C9 enzymes of the hepatic cytochrome P450 system – one reason for the wide variability in elimination [Werner et al., 2002]. It appears to inhibit CYP2D6, this may be the cause for interactions with beta blockers and psychoactive drugs. 99% of an administered dose is excreted by the biliary route and in the feces. In patients with moderately impaired hepatic function (serum albumin 25–35 g/L) the celecoxib dose should be reduced by one half. Celecoxib should not be used in patients with severe renal impairment.

Rofecoxib

Rofecoxib was introduced in the USA and Germany in 1999. Like celecoxib, this COX-2 inhibitor is approved for the treatment of activated osteoarthritis and rheumatoid arthritis. At 35, the COX-2 selectivity is higher than that of celecoxib [Riendeau et al., 2001]. Rofecoxib is readily and completely absorbed. Peak plasma concentration is reached after 2–3 hours and is unaffected by food intake. The elimination half-life is 17 hours. Rofecoxib is almost completely metabolized largely independent of the hepatic cytochrome P450 system. The metabolites are excreted predominantly by the kidneys.

Assessment of the potential efficacy and adverse effects of celecoxib and rofecoxib

The two COX-2 inhibitors have meanwhile been tested in numerous clinical trials for efficacy and safety in the treatment of osteoarthritis and rheumatoid arthritis. These included two large-scale randomized studies to investigate the gastrointestinal safety of the products in more than

8000 patients. In the CLASS trial (Celecoxib Long-term Arthritis Safety Study), celecoxib was compared to conventional NSAIDs (diclofenac or ibuprofen) in patients with osteoarthritis or rheumatoid arthritis. The VIGOR study (Vioxx Gastrointestinal Outcomes Research) included only patients with rheumatoid arthritis and compared rofecoxib to naproxen.

Efficacy. According to the available results, both specific COX-2 inhibitors have good analgesic and (somewhat less good) anti-inflammatory efficacy that is comparable, but not superior, to that of the other NSAIDs.

Gastrointestinal tolerance. The COX-2 inhibitors reduce the risk of severe gastrointestinal complications such as bleeding, perforation, and obstruction by one half. Thus the number of such events in the VIGOR study was 0.6 per 100 patient-years with rofecoxib and 1.4 per 100 patient-years with naproxen [Bombardier et al., 2000]. In the CLASS trial the corresponding figures were 2.08 events per 100 patient-years for celecoxib and 3.54 events per 100 patient-years for the comparator NSAIDs (ibuprofen or diclofenac) [Silverstein et al., 2000]. Both differences were statistically significant. However, the calculations for celecoxib are based only on the results from the first six months of the study; the complete one-year follow-up data were submitted only to the FDA and show no confirmed superiority of celecoxib. In any case, the figures presented make it clear that the occurrence of severe gastrointestinal complications cannot be ruled out with COX-2 inhibitors. Hence, not all high-risk patients benefit from treatment with a COX-2 inhibitor.

The general gastrointestinal tolerability of coxibs is better than that of conventional NSAIDs but poorer than that of, for example, acetaminophen. However, such "banal" side effects as abdominal pain, dyspepsia, nausea, and diarrhea are what prompt patients to discontinue treatment with NSAIDs in clinical practice. In the CLASS trial 14.4% of the patients treated with celecoxib reported dyspeptic symptoms (16.1% with naproxen) and 9.7% abdominal pain (13.1% with naproxen); in total 31.4% of the patients taking celecoxib (36.8% of those taking ibuprofen/diclofenac) had gastrointestinal side effects. In a 24-week study with osteoarthritis patients 8.3% and 9.5% of the patients receiving 25 and 50 mg rofecoxib daily, respectively, had abdominal pain. The rate in the ibuprofen group was 7.6% [Laine et al., 1999].

It also remains to be clarified whether coxibs impair healing of existing gastroduodenal ulcers. This could occur if a patient is switched from a conventional NSAID to as coxib. Increased expression of COX-2 has been found around the edge of ulcers, and COX-2 inhibitors were found to delay ulcer healing in mice [Mizuno et al., 1997]. However, unambiguous clinical evidence of such an effect has not yet been found.

Cardiovascular side effects. In view of the findings of the VIGOR study it has been proposed that COX-2 inhibitors may increase the risk of severe thrombotic events such as myocardial infarction, unstable angina, cardiac arrest, or ischemic stroke [Mukherjee et al., 2001]. The published data indicate an increased myocardial infarction rate in patients who, despite pre-existing cardiovascular disease, do not take acetylsalicylic acid concurrently with rofecoxib [Bombardier et al., 2000]. This phenomenon could be explained by the fact that COX-2 inhibitors inhibit vascular prostacyclins but not the antiplatelet eicosanoids, which are synthesized by COX-1. This could lead to an imbalance between pro- and antithrombotic eicosanoids. In the CLASS trial no such overhang of cardiovascular events was observed for celecoxib in comparison to ibuprofen or diclofenac (which have weaker antiplatelet activity than naproxen [White et al., 2002]. The results of the VIGOR study could therefore also be due to a protective effect of naproxen or to chance. Further prospective studies are required before a definitive assessment can be made.

It is conceivable that the hypertensive activity of the COX-2 inhibitors leads to an increased cardiovascular risk. Thus in the VIGOR study rofecoxib increased systolic blood pressure by 4.6 mmHg and diastolic blood pressure by 1.7 mmHg (naproxen: 1.0 and 0.1 mmHg, respectively) [Mukherjee et al., 2001] – a rise that is certainly within the clinically relevant range.

Nephrotoxicity. According to the available clinical and experimental data, renal function is affected no less by the selective COX-2 inhibitors than by conventional NSAIDs [Komers et al., 2001]. They selective COX-2 inhibitors can cause sodium, potassium, and water retention as well as elevated blood pressure. These side effects are especially marked in patients with volume and/or sodium depletion. In a short-term randomized study on healthy elderly volunteers (60–80 years) who received a low-salt diet, the influence of rofecoxib on renal function was comparable to that of indomethacin. In both groups glomerular filtration rate fell by approximately 12% [Swan et al., 2000]. In another study celecoxib caused the same salt and water retention as naproxen under conditions of salt restriction [Rossat et al., 1999]. In addition, cases of heart failure and acute renal failure were documented in high-risk patients on rofecoxib and celecoxib [Perazella and Tray, 2001]. Schwartz et al. (2002) showed that all renal effects of naproxen are also associated with celecoxib and rofecoxib. Deviations resulted only from the different durations of action of the drugs. Thus, the same precautions and contraindications that apply to conventional NSAIDs also apply to the selective COX-2 inhibitors.

Conclusions

Contrary to earlier expectations, the isoenzyme COX-2 is expressed in numerous cell systems and organs, even under physiologic conditions, where it evidently performs complex functions. In order to reliably assess the safety of the coxibs, extensive monitoring of patients will be required in future studies. More importantly, though, controlled studies are needed in order to evaluate the benefits and risks of these drugs in high-risk patients with renal disease, hypertension, cardiovascular disease, or heart failure. Special attention must also be paid to the reproductive system, endothelial functions, and wound healing. On the other hand, interesting new indications are emerging for the specific COX-2 inhibitors, e.g. in various tumors and Alzheimer's disease. Corresponding studies are already underway [Hinz und Brune, 2002].

Antipyretic analgesics without anti-inflammatory activity

Acetaminophen

Acetaminophen (paracetamol) is one of the most widely used drugs in the world. It exhibits good antipyretic and analgesic but no appreciable anti-inflammatory activity. Accordingly, the chief indications for acetaminophen are fever and mild to moderate pain. Even in severe pain treated with opiates, the analgesic effect can be enhanced by additionally administering acetaminophen (or NSAID). Thanks to its excellent safety profile, acetaminophen is considered to be the drug of first choice in children, pregnant women, and the elderly for the treatment of uncomplicated headache, osteoarthritis, and noninflammatory pain of the musculoskeletal system. Acetaminophen is particularly suitable for the treatment of patients for whom NSAIDs are contraindicated, e.g. due to acetylsalicylic acid asthma or a high risk of gastrointestinal complications. However, at the approved doses the efficacy of acetaminophen is often inadequate. In such cases other drugs must be used; in no circumstances should the dose be increased, as this could result in acute liver failure!

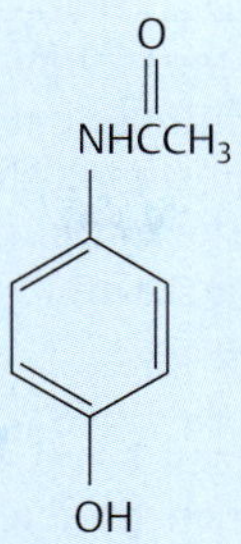

Paracetamol

Acetaminophen is the active metabolite of phenacetin, which has been withdrawn from the market due to its nephrotoxicity (interstitial nephritis). Acetaminophen is rapidly and completely absorbed from the gastrointestinal tract and reaches peak plasma concentrations after approximately 30–60 minutes. The mean plasma half-life is around two hours. Acetaminophen is metabolized in the liver and is renally excreted, chiefly in the form of glucuronide and sulfate. Its metabolism is affected to a clinically relevant degree and its half-life prolonged only in severe acute or chronic hepatic impairment.

Despite extensive research, the mechanism of action of acetaminophen has not yet been satisfactorily elucidated. Acetaminophen is only a weak inhibitor of the two isoenzymes COX-1 and COX-2. Recently inhibition of a splice variant of COX-1, termed COX-3, has been claimed [Chandrasekharan et al., 2002]. Contrary to earlier hypotheses, it is now assumed that the action of acetaminophen relies not on peripheral mechanisms but on the inhibition of prostaglandin biosynthesis in the hypothalamus and spinal cord. The central action hypothesis is supported by numerous facts: Acetaminophen does not affect platelet aggregation of hemostasis and has a low plasma binding rate. The molecule occurs in undissociated form at physiologic pH values and readily crosses the blood-brain barrier.

It has been found in recent experiments on rats that intraperitoneally administered acetaminophen inhibits spinal PGE_2 release in the posterior horn of the spinal cord following peripheral noxious stimulation [Muth-Selbach et al., 1999]. Since the excretion of prostanoids in the animals' urine did not change, the antinociceptive effect does not appear to be due to inhibition of peripheral prostaglandin synthesis.

The recommended maximum daily dose of acetaminophen is between 2 and 4 g. In this dosage range acetaminophen produces hardly any side effects. Notably, the typical toxicity of NSAIDs is absent. In rare cases renal impairment has occurred following long-term use of therapeutic doses. Rash and severe hypersensitivity reactions are extremely rare. However, the therapeutic window for acetaminophen is narrow. Thus, liver functional disturbances and even irreversible liver cell necroses and hepatic coma may occur after high doses of > 4 to 7 g daily. In cases of overdosage the SH-group donor N-acetylcysteine has proved a useful antidote, provided that it is given within 16 hours of the overdose. It should be noted that microsomal enzyme inductors such as phenobarbital enhance the hepatotoxicity of acetaminophen. Patients with a high alcohol consumption also appear to be at increased risk. The dose must be reduced in patients with renal impairment; patients with preexisting liver damage and chronic alcoholics should not receive acetaminophen. Although acetaminophen has no direct effect on platelet aggregation or blood clotting, it can interact with warfarin to prolong bleeding time.

Dipyrone

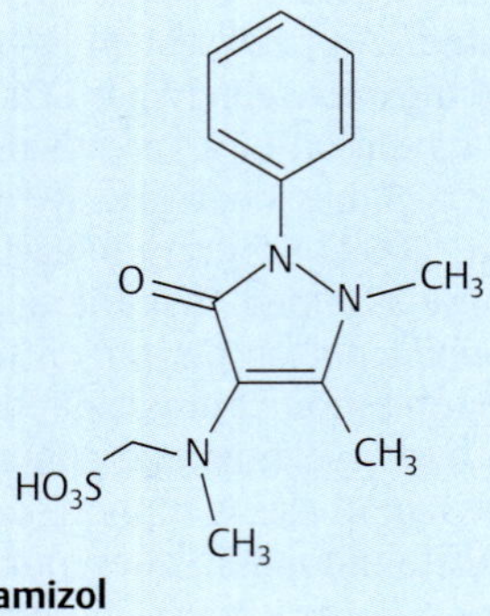

Metamizol

Dipyrone (metamizol) is a prodrug of the phenazone derivative methylaminophenazone (a weak base). It has been marketed in Germany since 1921. In terms of its analgesic and antipyretic effect it is superior to both acetylsalicylic acid and acetaminophen. It also has a spasmolytic effect on the smooth muscle of the gastrointestinal and urinary tracts. Since it is readily soluble in water, dipyrone can also be given intravenously but should then be injected slowly to avoid the risk of shock reactions. Depending on the dosage form, peak plasma levels are reached after about 20 minutes (drops) to one hour (tablets) after oral administration. The maximum daily dose is 4 g. Despite unselective COX-1 and COX-2 inhibition, dipyrone is not associated with gastrointestinal damage, fluid retention, or inhibition of blood clotting. The risk of agranulocytosis is reported to be one in one million. If GM-CSF is given in time, the hematologic changes are reversible. Very rarely, severe allergic skin reactions and hypotension can also occur. Overall, however, the risk of a fatal adverse reaction with dipyrone is estimated to be less than that associated with conventional NSAIDs (gastrointestinal bleeding).

3.2 Opiates/Opioids

In the series from weak to potent agents, the narcotic analgesics represent the last escalation stage in the treatment of acute and chronic persistent pain. They are used when the response to NSAIDs and analgesics without an anti-inflammatory component is no longer satisfactory.

The narcotic analgesics form a highly heterogeneous group of substances comprising plant alkaloids (the opiates morphine, codeine, etc.), a series of synthetic compounds (the opioids), and a large number of naturally occurring peptides (β-endorphins, enkephalins, dynorphins) occurring in the central nervous system of humans and other mammals. The pharmacologic action of the exogenous opiates/opioids that can be therapeutically used as analgesics derives from the fact that they simulate the action of endogenous chemical messengers at enkephalin receptors: They are all enkephalinergic (partial) agonists.

In addition to their analgesic effects, the opioids have a broad range of other desirable and undesirable effects, though there may be differences between individual synthetic opioids and morphine. The central suppressive activity of the opioids includes, in addition to analgesia, respiratory depressant, sedative, anxiolytic, antitussive, and antiemetic effects. The opioids also act as euphoriants (central activating effect). The most important peripheral effects include constipation, urinary retention, cholestasis, tocolysis, and hypotension.

Two other common properties of the opioids become problematic only during long-term use. First, the body develops tolerance to the central effects (but not to the peripheral effects) of the opioids. This means that the analgesic effect can decline in the course of treatment and has to be compensated for by dose escalation. Second, regular use leads to physical (and to a lesser extent psychological) dependence. Both problems are rare in chronic pain patients receiving a constant opiate/opioid dose.

The opiates/opioids can be distinguished on the basis of their analgesic strength:

- **Weak opiates/opioids** include codeine, dextropropoxyphene, tilidine (+ naloxone), and tramadol.
- **Strong opiates/opioids** are buprenorphine, fentanyl, levomethadone, morphine, pentazocine, pethidine, and piritramide.

Common to all opioids is a basic pK value. Protein binding varies between < 10% and 90%, depending on the lipophilic character of the molecule. There are substantial differences in terms of oral availability and elimination half-life. **Dextropropoxyphene** (Develin® delayed release) is rapidly absorbed and, with a mean half-life of 12 hours, is given twice daily (morning and evening, 150 mg to max. 300 mg b.i.d.). **Tramadol** can be a sensible adjuvant to long-term treatment with NSAIDs in the elderly, as it does not have the latter's cardiovascular side effects (exacerbation of hypertension and heart failure), nor does it cause gastrointestinal ulcers [Katz, 1996]. With tramadol the typical opioid-related side effects such as respiratory depression and constipation are of little clinical relevance, and the dependence potential is low. Although nausea may occur in the initial stage of treatment, it can be lessened by slowly increasing (titrating) the dose. For chronic pain a sustained-release formulation (e.g. Tramal® long) can be used, which only has to be taken twice daily (100 – 200 mg in the morning and evening).

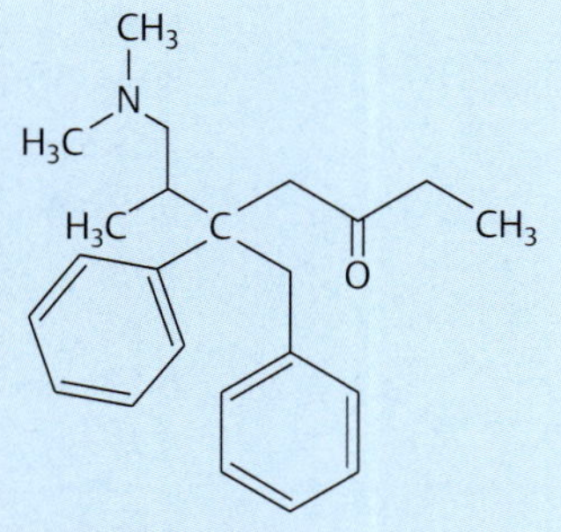

Dextropropoxyphen

Only in rare exceptional cases do potent opiates/opioids play a role in the treatment of pain of the musculoskeletal system (except tumor pain).

3.3 Glucocorticoids

Glucocorticoids are the most effective anti-inflammatory drugs currently available. They have no direct analgesic activity. The pain relief experienced by arthritis patients on corticosteroids is due to a reduction of inflammatory activity and inhibition of COX-2 formation. The use of corticosteroids usually has no justification in purely degenerative arthritic pain.

In addition to suppressing inflammation, glucocorticoids have numerous other pharmacologically useful effects. They are, for example,

- antiallergic
- antiproliferative
- antiexudative and
- immunosuppressant.

The mechanism of action is correspondingly complex and is not yet fully understood. In simplified terms, it may be assumed that corticosteroids diffuse passively through the cell membrane and bind to specific cytoplasmic receptors that occur in nearly all cells of the body. The steroid-receptor complex migrates into the nucleus, where it induces the transcription of mRNAs that code for numerous proteins. As a result, the synthesis of proinflammatory cytokines such as IL-1, IL-6, and TNF-α is reduced. Another mechanism that contributes to the anti-inflammatory activity of glucocorticoids is inhibition of the expression of inducible cyclooxygenase-2 (COX-2). This reduces the synthesis of prostaglandins. All these genome-mediated effects have a late onset and reach their peak only after 1 – 8 hours. In addition, there are also rapid steroid-induced effects. If, following high doses of a glucocorticoid (e.g. 200 – 300 mg prednisolone) all the corticosteroids receptors are occupied, unspecific nongenomic effects occur within seconds to minutes. These can be explained in terms of physicochemical interactions with cell membranes and include, for example, permeability changes in vascular endothelial cells.

Although glucocorticoids with markedly greater anti-inflammatory and weaker mineralocorticoid effects have been developed by synthesizing derivatives of the endogenous adrenal cortical hormones cortisone and cortisol, it has not been possible to fully eliminate the sometimes severe adverse effects (Table 3.**1**). Patients therefore have to be closely and carefully monitored especially during long-term therapy with glucocorticoids:

- **Before treatment is initiated** active/acute infections must be ruled out.
- **Every two weeks** (in the case of low-dose long-term therapy every 1 – 2 months) the patient should be asked about and examined for the occurrence of side effects (including measurement of vital functions).
- **Every three months the** blood sedimentation rate, blood cell counts, urinary sediment, and blood sugar should be checked, and the patient should undergo an ophthalmologic examination.
- **Every six months** a cardiologic examination and assay of lipid levels should be performed.

The actual adverse-effect risk associated with glucocorticoid therapy depends on the nature of the drug, the dose, the duration of treatment, any coadministered medication, and patient-specific factors (gender, age, concurrent diseases, etc.). Today **prednisone** and **prednisolone** as well as their nonfluorated derivatives are used in systemic therapy. Usually having a longer elimination half-life, the fluorated substances bring about greater suppression of the adrenal regulation circuit, so that their use is largely limited to topical treatment. Table 3.**2** shows the equivalent doses for various glucocorticoids.

Special therapeutic forms have been developed in order to minimize the adverse-effect risk:

- **High-dose intravenous shock therapy.** In acute and potentially threatening conditions (e.g. severe systemic disease, complication of giant-cell arteritis, severe episodes of rheumatoid arthritis, etc.) high to extremely high doses are administered for short periods (in a hospital setting!): 500 – 1000 mg prednisolone as an i.v. infusion on one to five successive days, possibly repeated every month; in the case of joint changes continuous low-

Table 3.**1** Adverse effects of anti-inflammatory therapy with glucocorticoids

Adverse Effect
▪ Suppression of endogenous cortisol production (adrenocortical contraction)
▪ Cushing's syndrome in long-term high-dose therapy (moon face, adiposity of the trunk, skin and muscular wasting)
▪ Inhibition of protein synthesis (catabol)
▪ Osteoporosis (suppression of osteoblasts, stimulation of osteoclasts, inhibition of calcium absorption and renal calcium reabsorption), and osteonecrosis
▪ Growth retardation in children
▪ Menstruation and potency disturbances
▪ Hirsutism
▪ Prodiabetic effects (reduction of glucose uptake into cells, increased gluconeogenesis)
▪ Psychotropic effects (acute mood and drive swings, psychoses)
▪ Inhibition of cellular immune defense (increased infection risk)
▪ Enhanced ulcerogenic effects of NSAIDs
▪ Water and sodium retention, increased potassium excretion (edema, hypertension, exacerbation of heart failure)
▪ Pancreatitis
▪ Cataract and glaucoma

Table 3.**2** Equivalent doses of the most important glucocorticoids [after Miehle, 2000]

Glucocorticoid	Dose
For comparison: cortisol	**25 mg**
Prednisone	5 mg
Prednisolone	5 mg
Prednylidene	6 mg
6-methylprednisolone	4 mg
Cloprednol	2.5 – 5 mg
Deflazacort	6 – 9 mg
Fluocortolone	5 mg
Triamcinolone	4 mg
Dexamethasone	0.75 mg
Betamethasone	0.75 mg

dose oral corticosteroid therapy in the interval. Shock therapy can also be given orally with prednisolone 1 – 1.5 mg/kg daily.

– **"Low-dose" therapy.** Chronic diseases requiring long-term therapy are treated with the smallest corticosteroid dose that is still effective. This dose needs to be individually titrated. To this end, the initial dose is reduced gradually – sometimes over several months – in increments of 1 mg and later 0.5 mg prednisolone daily. A daily dose of 5 mg prednisolone is evidently sufficiently effective in most inflammatory rheumatic diseases. If possible, adults should receive 30 mg or less daily taken in a single dose in the morning (if this proves insufficient for severe symptoms ⅔ in the morning and ⅓ in the afternoon). Growing children should not receive corticosteroids more often than once every 48 hours (alternating therapy).

Table 3.**3** Onset of action of various disease-modifying drugs

After several days
▪ Etanercept
After 1 – 3 months
▪ Leflunomide
▪ Methotrexate
▪ Cyclosporin
▪ Cyclophosphamide
▪ Sulfasalazine
▪ Azathioprine
After 4 to > 6 months
▪ Chloroquine
▪ Hydroxychloroquine
▪ Aurothioglucose
▪ Auranofin
▪ D-penicillamine
▪ OM-8980 (Subreum)?

Whenever possible corticosteroids should be used **locally** (possibly also **intra-articularly**). This form of administration permits lasting therapeutic success and largely avoids systemic side effects. However, the drug used should be poorly soluble to produce effective intra-articular but low systemic concentrations. It is particularly advisable, owing to the possibility of crystal-induced irritation, to use products with modern formulations, e.g. lipid microspheres.

Because of the significantly increased risk of ulceration, **NSAIDs** should **not** be given in combination with corticosteroid therapy. During long-term treatment with corticosteroids every patient should practice **osteoporosis prophylaxis:** a daily calcium intake of 1000 – 1500 mg (in elderly patients with poor nutrition or little exposure to the sun additionally 400 – 1000 IU of vitamin D), physical exercise, and in postmenopausal women hormone replacement. In high-risk patients and/or patients with pre-existing osteoporosis further therapeutic measures are called for (bisphosphonates).

3.4 Disease-modifying anti-rheumatic drugs and biologicals

The disease-modifying anti-rheumatic drugs (DMARDs), also known as slow-acting anti-rheumatic drugs (SAARDs), do not live up to the claim that they fundamentally influence the pathogenesis of the rheumatic diseases for which they are used (usually rheumatoid arthritis) or are even curative. However, they can slow the progression of the disease in the short or mid and sometimes even in the long term, and occasionally bring about surprising improvements in symptoms and laboratory parameters, including lasting complete remission (biologicals). Based on today's understanding, SAARD therapy should therefore be used as soon as possible after diagnosis in order to halt joint destruction.

Since the SAARDs do not have direct anti-inflammatory and analgesic effects and their desired effects are often not felt for weeks to months (Table 3.**3**), they usually have to be combined with NSAIDs and/or glucocorticoids.

Unlike other antirheumatic drugs, the effects of the SAARDs persist (with some exceptions) for some time after they have been discontinued. However, withdrawal always carries a risk: Even after successful long-term therapy there is no guarantee that the patient will respond to the same SAARD when treatment is resumed. For this reason, after long-term partial or full remission a cautious attempt should be made to reduce the dosage.

If no improvement is discernible after around six months' treatment with an SAARD, the therapeutic attempt should be abandoned and the patient should be put on another drug.

The SAARDs include a number chemically highly heterogeneous substances, some of which are associated with serious side effects. Disease-modifying therapy therefore always presupposes cooperation on the part of the patients and close monitoring of clinical signs and laboratory parameters. As for the mode of action of many of the SAARDs, only rudimentary knowledge is available. The choice of agent depends on the inflammatory activity and the prognosis. Although in principle all the SAARDs can be used in rheumatoid arthritis, certain drugs are preferentially used in specific clinical pictures, e.g. methotrexate and sulfasalazine in chronic reactive arthritis and methotrexate, chloroquine/hydroxychloroquine, and azathioprine in collagen diseases.

Antimalarial agents

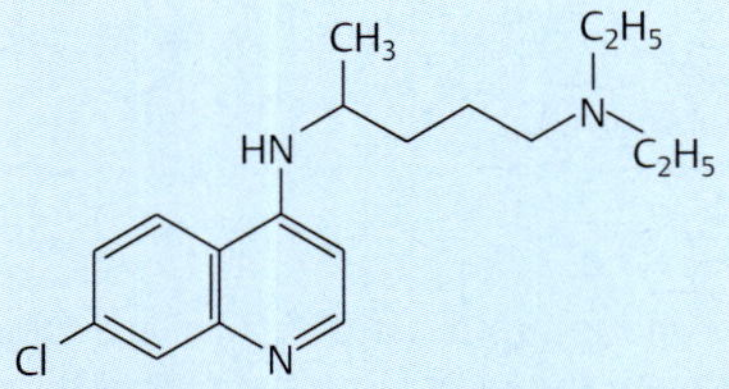

Chloroquine

Drugs: Chloroquine, hydroxychloroquine.

Evaluation: The safest available SAARD but not very effective. Success rate approximately 25% in rheumatoid arthritis.

Mechanisms of action: Accumulation in lysosomes and inhibition of antigen processing (reduced antibody production, inhibition of natural killer cells, reduced release of IL-1, IL-2, and TNF-α). Immunosuppression via several mechanisms.

Pharmacokinetics: Rapid and complete absorption. High accumulation in some blood cells, internal organs, and the eyes (retina, uvea). Terminal half-life > 40 days due to slow depletion of tissue stores. Slow elimination, 40–70% of the substance being excreted unchanged in the urine, the rest via the liver and biliary tract with the feces.

Indications: Lupus erythematosus without serious organ involvement, e.g. cutaneous discoid lupus erythematosus (possibly in combination with an immunosuppressant such as azathioprine); rheumatoid arthritis, especially less active early cases.

Onset of action: Long (up to six months).

Dosage: Chloroquine 250 mg (max. 4 mg/kg), hydroxychloroquine 200–300 mg (max. 6 mg/kg).

Adverse effects (selection): *Common:* gastrointestinal effects (nausea, anorexia, diarrhea); *rare:* dermatologic (rash, pigment anomalies, pruritus), cardiologic effects (hypotension, negative T-waves in the ECG), neurologic effects (headache, dizziness, paresthesia, sleep disturbances, neuromyopathy, seizures), ophthalmologic effects (accommodation disturbances, corneal inclusions, photosensitivity, disturbances of color vision); *very rare:* irreversible retinopathy (early symptom = defective red vision), hematologic effects (thrombocytopenia, agranulocytosis, pancytopenia).

Monitoring: An ophthalmologic examination should be performed before treatment is initiated. Monitoring every two weeks initially and then after the fourth month every two months (history-taking and laboratory tests for adverse effects); An ophthalmologic examination should be repeated every 4–6 months.

Sulfasalazine

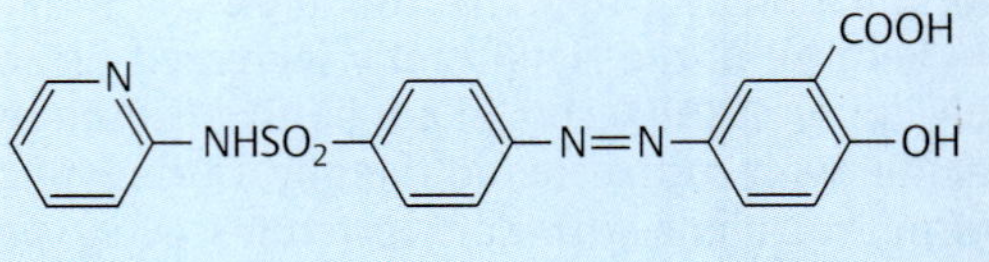

Sulfasalazine

Evaluation: Good success in rheumatoid arthritis during the first two years of treatment. A long-term effect on radiologically confirmed progression is doubtful.

Mechanisms of action: Immunomodulating effect by reducing immunoglobulin levels (especially IgA), inhibition of mitogen-stimulating lymphocyte proliferation, and reduction of various cytokines. Inhibition of IgE-induced mast-cell degranulation and proliferation of endothelial cells. Anti-inflammatory action via inhibition of leukotriene B_4 production.

Pharmacokinetics: 10–20% of an orally administered dose is absorbed. Some enters the enterohepatic circulation. After biliary excretion the drug is split in the colon into the two active substances sulfapyridine and 5-aminoacetylsalicylic acid. Plasma half-life between 5.5 and 15 hours depending on the genetic acetylation phenotype.

Indications: Early stages of rheumatoid arthritis (mild to moderate activity), chronic reactive arthritis, spondylarthritis with peripheral joint involvement.

Onset of action: Moderately long (2 – 3 months).

Dosage: Initial therapy with 500 mg daily, increased at weekly intervals in 500-mg-increments to 2 g daily (maximum 3 g daily).

Adverse effects (selection): *Common:* gastrointestinal effects (nausea, vomiting, dyspepsia), central nervous effects (headache, fatigue, confusion), allergies, dermatologic effects (rash, pruritus); *rare:* elevated hepatic enzymes, hematologic effects (leukopenia, thrombocytopenia, elevated MCV); *very rare:* severe adverse reactions such as Stevens-Johnson or Lyell's syndrome, aplastic anemia, agranulocytosis; liver, CNS, kidney damage.

Monitoring: Initially every two weeks, from the 4th to 6th month every four weeks, and then every three months thereafter (history-taking and laboratory tests for adverse effects).

Oral gold therapy

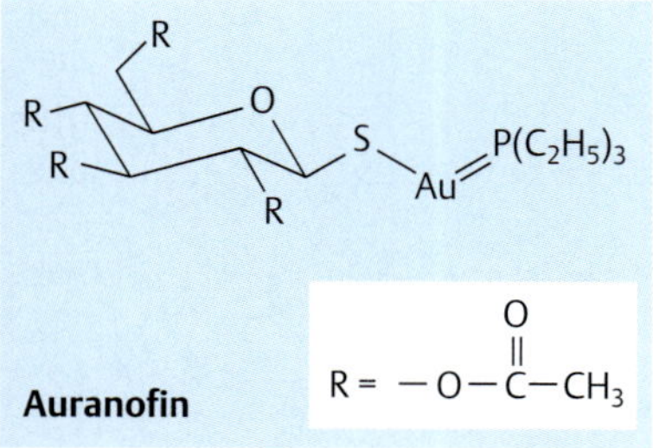

Auranofin

Drug: Auranofin

Evaluation: Less effective than parenteral gold, somewhat more effective than the antimalarial drugs (success rate 30 – 50 % in rheumatoid arthritis).

Mechanisms of action: Inhibition of cellular and humoral immune processes, inhibition of prostaglandin activity and platelet aggregation, binds oxygen radicals.

Pharmacokinetics: 25 % of an oral dose is absorbed. Plasma binding (especially to serum iron) 60 %. Plasma half-life 11 – 31 days, total body half-life 81 days (retention of approximately 59 mg gold after 6 months' treatment). 95 % excreted in the feces.

Indications: All cases of rheumatoid arthritis that are no longer treatable with antimalarial drugs as well as psoriatic arthritis and spondylarthritis with peripheral involvement of joints.

Onset of action: Long (approximately four months).

Dosage: Initially and as long-term therapy one to two 3-mg tablets daily; increase to three tablets daily (after 4 – 6 months) only if the patient fails to respond.

Adverse effects (selection): *Common:* gastrointestinal effects (diarrhea, nausea) and dermatologic effects (dermatitis, stomatitis, pruritus); *rare:* hematologic effects (granulocytopenia, thrombocytopenia, eosinophilia, anemia), pulmonary effects (bronchiolitis, pulmonary fibrosis), kidney damage.

Monitoring: Initially every two months. From the fourth month every four weeks (history-taking and laboratory tests for adverse effects).

Parenteral gold therapy

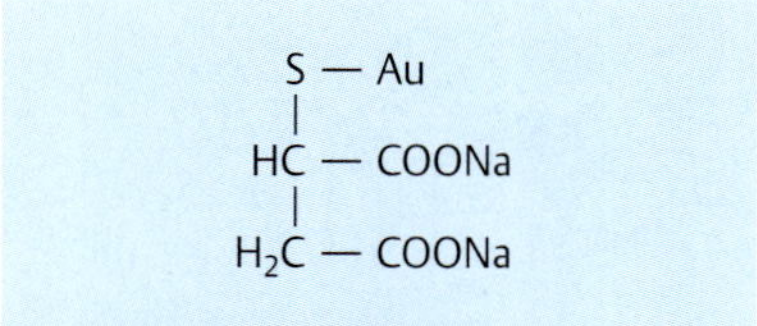

Sodium aurothiomalate

Drug: Sodium aurothiomalate

Evaluation: Better efficacy, but also a higher adverse-effect rate than with the antimalarial drugs. Confirmed therapeutic value in rheumatoid arthritis (response rate approximately 65%).

Mechanisms of action: Immunomodulating and anti-inflammatory action, similar to oral gold salts.

Pharmacokinetics: Stable gold levels of 300–400 µg/dl are reached 6–8 weeks after weekly i.m. injections, during maintenance therapy 75–125 µg/dl. 80–90% of each i.m. gold dose is excreted by the kidneys, the rest in the feces. Gold salts have special affinity for inflamed tissues, e.g. the synovium.

Indications: Like oral gold therapy. Because of the risk of sensitization parenteral gold is unsuitable in lupoid forms of rheumatoid arthritis or in systemic lupus erythematosus.

Onset of action: Long (3–6 months).

Dosage: Initial test dose of 10 mg i.m. (allergy testing), one week later 20 mg i.m. (saturation), then 50 mg i.m. once weekly up to the 20th week, followed by maintenance therapy with 50 mg i.m. every 2–4 weeks depending on the disease activity.

Adverse effects (selection): Similar to oral gold therapy; in addition the common (harmless) occurrence of deposits in the cornea and lens.

Monitoring: Initially every two months. From the fourth month every four weeks (history-taking and laboratory tests for adverse effects).

D-penicillamine

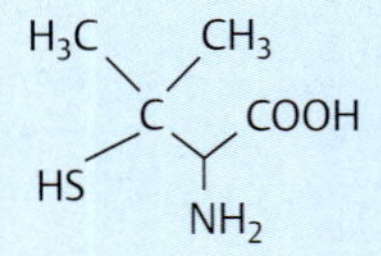

Penicillamine

Evaluation: At present only a second choice drug due to high toxicity and very late onset of action. Overall poorer risk-benefit relationship than with other SAARDs.

Mechanisms of action: Dissociates and reduces circulating immune complexes, accelerates cytokine degradation, inhibits T-cell functions, antiangiogenetic and antifibrotic action.

Pharmacokinetics: Absorption rate 40–70% (reduced in the presence of gastrointestinal disease). Plasma half-life 70–100 hours. The drug accumulates in collagen-rich tissues. 75–80% of metabolites are eliminated renally, the rest in the feces.

Indications: Similar to gold therapy. Because of its antifibrotic effect D-penicillamine is also useful in progressive systemic sclerosis.

Onset of action: Long (3–6 months).

Dosage: Slow dose escalation with 150 mg daily in the first two weeks, 300 mg daily in the third and fourth weeks, 450 mg daily in the fifth and sixth weeks, and 600 mg daily up to the 16th week. If the response is unsatisfactory, the dose can be further increased. The maintenance dose is approximately 450–600 mg daily.

Adverse effects (selection): *Common:* dermatologic effects (rash, stomatitis, pruritus), gastrointestinal effects (nausea, vomiting), thrombocytopenia, myasthenia, proteinuria, hypogeusia/ageusia. Numerous other rarer adverse effects.

Monitoring: Initially every two months. From the fourth month every four weeks (history-taking and laboratory tests for adverse effects).

Methotrexate

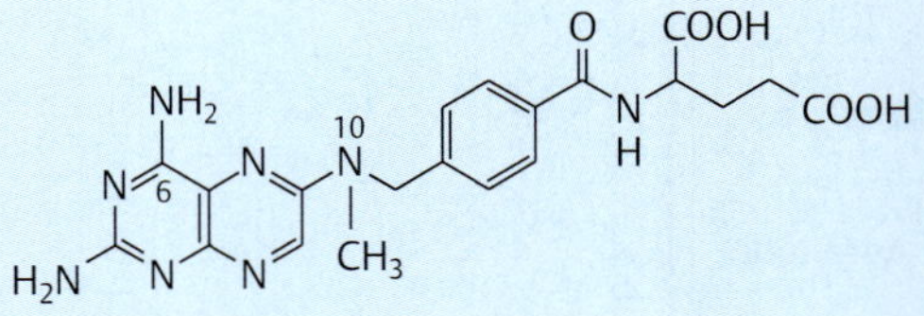

Methotrexate

Evaluation: An atypical SAARD (no effect beyond administration, an inconsistent effect on parameters of inflammation) with rapid onset of action and efficacy in pathogenetically very different diseases. Long-term treatment is possible thanks to relatively good compliance.

Mechanisms of action: Antimetabolite and antiproliferative activity via suppression of tetrahydrofolic acid production. It is unclear if this mechanism alone is responsible for the drug's efficacy in rheumatoid arthritis. More important appear to be effects on cytokines (e.g. IL-1), anti-inflammatory activity due to inhibition of neutrophil chemotaxis and leukocyte adhesion, and antiangiogenetic activity.

Pharmacokinetics: Mean bioavailability 70% following oral and parental administration, but with large interindividual variation (reason for occasional nonresponse in oral therapy?). The elimination half-life is 6–8 hours, sometimes significantly longer. Variable enterohepatic recirculation.

Indications: Rheumatoid arthritis in adults, juvenile chronic arthritis, psoriatic arthritis, and psoriasis, increasingly also other rheumatic diseases and systemic lupus erythematosus.

Onset of action: Short (4–8 weeks).

Dosage: Once weekly in individually titrated doses of 7.5 to 25 mg, depending on body weight, usually orally but also i.v., i.m., or s.c. if there are compliance problems or marked disease activity.

Adverse effects (selection): *Common:* dermatologic effects (stomatitis, alopecia), gastrointestinal effects (nausea, vomiting), elevated transaminases. Teratogenic effect, increased susceptibility to infection. Numerous other rarer adverse effects.

Monitoring: After two and four weeks and monthly thereafter.

Azathioprine

Evaluation: Effective SAARD in specific indications.

Mechanisms of action: Predominantly immunosuppressant (T, B lymphocytes, killer cells); inhibits the activity of IL-6.

Pharmacokinetics: Approximately 88% of an oral dose is absorbed. The plasma half-life is 60–90 minutes. The metabolites are excreted chiefly by the kidneys.

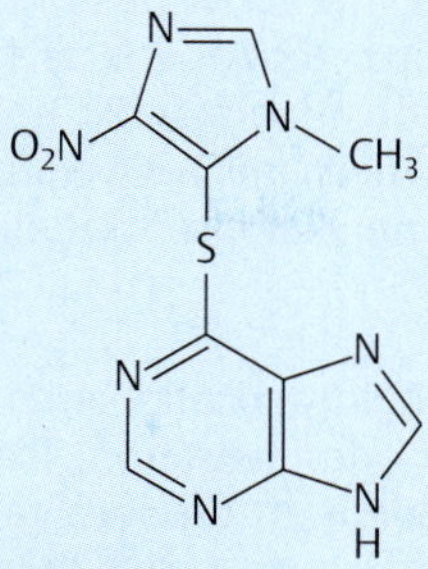

Azathioprine

Indications: Various collagen diseases, e.g. systemic lupus erythematosus, mixed collagenosis, primary Sjögren's syndrome, etc. Rheumatoid arthritis if other SAARDs are no longer effective, are poorly tolerated or are contraindicated as well as in highly active or malignant clinical pictures.

Onset of action: Relatively long (2–6 months).

Dosage: Individually titrated dose, best based on body weight, of 1.5–3 mg/kg daily (adults) or 2–3 mg/kg daily (children); in patients with renal impairment (creatinine clearance $<$ 20 mg/ml) the maximum dose is limited to 1.5 mg/kg.

Adverse effects (selection): *Common:* gastrointestinal effects (nausea, vomiting, diarrhea), hematologic effects (leukopenia, anemia), infections, drug fever. Numerous other rarer adverse effects.

Monitoring: Initially every 8 to 14 days, from the third month every four weeks.

Cyclophosphamide

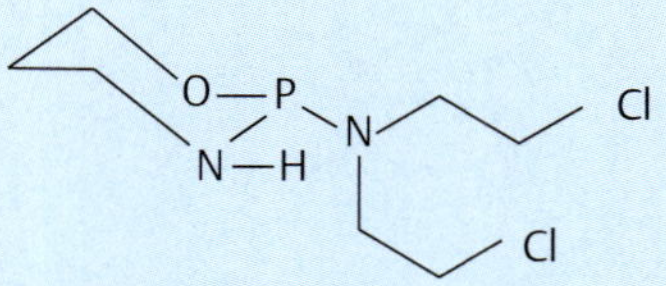

Cyclophosphamide

Evaluation: Effective drug in refractory cases of rheumatoid arthritis and systemic lupus erythematosus but, being carcinogenic, is suitable only as an emergency drug.

Mechanisms of action: The active metabolites alkylate DNA, resulting in cytotoxic effects. Numerous immunologic and inflammatory processes are influenced by this mechanism. Overall, cyclophosphamide has immunosuppressant and anti-inflammatory activity.

Pharmacokinetics: Rapid and almost complete absorption after oral administration. Excessive metabolism occurs chiefly in the liver (affected by, among other drugs, glucocorticoids, phenobarbital, and allopurinol). The plasma half-life is 2 – 10 hours. Only 20 % of the substance is excreted unchanged in the urine within 24 hours.

Indications: Acute forms of granulomatous vasculitis and polyarteritis nodosa (also in combination with a glucocorticoid); systemic lupus erythematosus with organ manifestations. In rheumatoid arthritis only as a backup drug or in the most severe cases with organ involvement.

Onset of action: Short (2 – 4 weeks in long-term therapy; in bolus therapy after the second to third bolus).

Dosage: In long-term oral therapy (the Fauci regimen) 1.0 to 4.0 mg/kg daily according to the leukocyte count (≥ 4000/µl) up to a cumulative maximum total dose of 50 g. In intravenous bolus therapy (the Austin regimen) 15 – 20 mg/kg every 3 – 4 weeks together with i.v. Mesna (in three divided doses after 0.4 and 8 hours) for cystitis prophylaxis.

Adverse effects (selection): *Common:* leukopenia (dose-dependent) and infections; permanent infertility and teratogenicity; markedly increased cancer risk.

Monitoring: In long-term therapy initially often. Later blood tests should be performed at least every four weeks. In bolus therapy blood tests should be performed 8 – 12 days after every treatment.

Cyclosporin

Evaluation: Not yet definitively possible; progress through the development of low-dose therapy and a dosage form with improved pharmacokinetics (Sandimmun® Optoral). Because of its chemosensitizing effect, cyclosporin is suitable for combination therapy. The effect does not exceed the administration of the drug.

Mechanisms of action: Immunosuppression through inhibition of T-helper cell activation; inhibits the synthesis of various cytokines and nuclear transcription factors, inhibits the expression of cytokine receptors and HOLA-DR antigens. Synergistic activity with hydroxychloroquine.

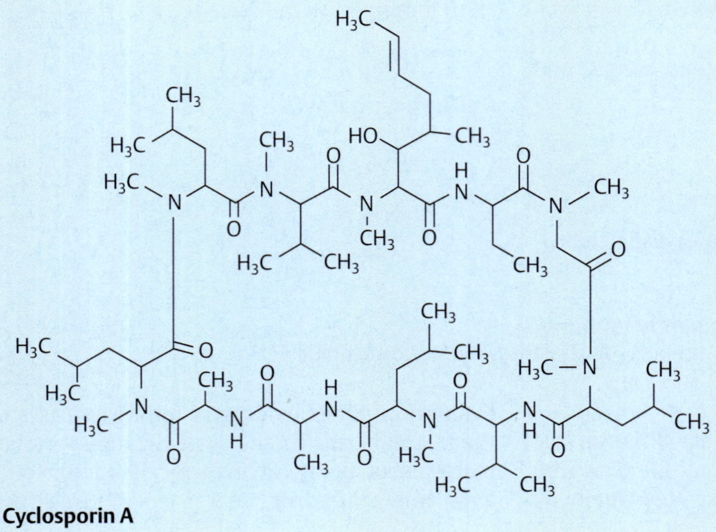

Cyclosporin A

Pharmacokinetics: Bioavailability at the start of treatment 4–26%, rising in the further course of treatment to as high as 50% (bioavailability of the new Sandimmun® Optoral nearly one third greater than that of Sandimmun®, also linear pharmacokinetics). Accumulates in tissue. Extensively metabolized in the liver (cytochrome P450) so that its pharmacokinetics may be affected by other drugs that compete for the same enzyme system. The elimination half-life is 6–20 hours. Elimination is predominantly by the biliary route.

Indications: Rheumatoid arthritis, psoriasis, fulminating anterior uveitis; even less experience in systemic lupus erythematosus and psoriatic arthritis.

Onset of action: Short (4–8 weeks).

Dosage: Initially 2.5–3 mg/kg daily. If no response is evident after 4–8 weeks, the dose is increased gradually to a maximum dose of 5 mg/kg daily. If there is still no response, the drug should be withdrawn slowly (due to a possible rebound effect).

Adverse effects (selection): *Common:* gastrointestinal effects (nausea, vomiting, diarrhea, liver function disturbances), dermatologic effects (hypertrichosis, gingival hyperplasia), nephrologic effects (renal impairment, hypertension), neurologic effects (tremor, fatigue, paresthesia). Numerous other rarer adverse effects.

Monitoring: Initially every 1–2 weeks, from the third month every four weeks.

Leflunomide

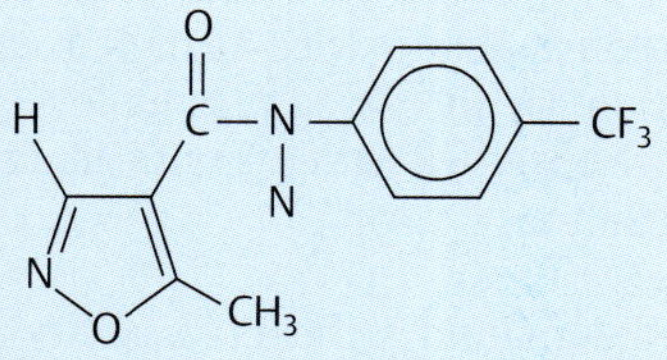

Leflunomide

Evaluation: Good efficacy (comparable to that of methotrexate and sulfasalazine) and adequate tolerance in rheumatoid arthritis. Clinical experience in combination therapy is still limited.

Mechanisms of action: Leflunomide is an isoxazole derivative with anti-inflammatory, antiproliferative, and immunomodulating activity. The primary effect is the selective inhibition of the *de novo* synthesis of pyrimidine ribonucleotides, which evidently chiefly affects the proliferation of activated autoimmune lymphocytes. The anti-inflammatory effect may be due to inhibition of IL-1, TNF-α, and nuclear factor NFκB.

Pharmacokinetics: Leflunomide is a prodrug that is rapidly and completely converted to an active metabolite following oral administration. The latter is almost completely bound to serum proteins. Half is eliminated in the bile, the other half by the kidneys. The elimination half-life is 10–30 days. The extent of accumulation is difficult to predict.

Indications: Rheumatoid arthritis if other SAARDs such as methotrexate and sulfasalazine prove ineffective or poorly tolerated.

Onset of action: Short (4–6 weeks). The effect may increase in the course of the following four to six months.

Dosage: Initial saturation with 100 mg once daily for three days, followed by maintenance therapy with 10–20 mg daily.

Adverse effects (selection): *Common:* hypertension (usually mild), elevated transaminase levels, allergic reactions, leukopenia, gastrointestinal effects (diarrhea, nausea, vomiting, anorexia, stomatitis), metabolic effects (weight loss, occasionally hypokalemia), neurologic effects (headache, dizziness, weakness, paresthesia), dermatologic effects (alopecia, eczema, dry skin); numerous *rare* adverse effects; *very rare:* agranulocytosis, Stevens-Johnson syndrome.

Monitoring: Initially every two weeks (ALAT, blood count). From the seventh month every eight weeks. The possibility of accumulation should be considered if diarrhea persists.

Infliximab

(See Fig. 4.8 for structure)

Evaluation: Because of the murine component in its molecule, infliximab can induce antibodies and should therefore be used only in combination with methotrexate. In the only randomized phase III study so far conducted, infliximab enhanced the effect of methotrexate. Experience outside clinical trials is still limited. Infliximab may be used only if the patient fails to respond to other (more cost-effective) SAARDs.

Mechanisms of action: Infliximab is a chimeric antibody whose constant region (Fc portion) consists of human IgG_1 and whose variable, antigen-binding region (Fab portion) is of murine origin. Infliximab specifically binds to TNF-α, leading via activation of the complement system to the lysis of TNF-α-expressing cells in inflamed joints and to suppression of TNF-α-triggered proinflammatory cytokines, e.g. IL-1, IL-6, and IL-8. Infliximab also inhibits the expression of endothelial adhesion molecules and thus the migration of leukocytes and normalizes C-reactive protein.

Pharmacokinetics: Infliximab is administered parenterally. In the dosage range of 1 to 20 mg/kg it exhibits linear pharmacokinetics. The small distribution volume of 3–4 liters indicates that infliximab remains largely sequestered within the vascular compartment. The terminal elimination half-life is in the range of 8 to 9.5 days. The elimination routes are still unclarified.

Indications: Used in combination with methotrexate for the treatment of rheumatoid arthritis that has responded inadequately to other SAARDs, including methotrexate. Infliximab is contraindicated in tuberculosis and other severe infections as well as in moderate to severe heart failure.

Onset of action: Very short (from two weeks).

Dosage: Intravenous infusions of 3 mg/kg over two hours in weeks 0, 2, and 6, then every eight weeks.

Adverse effects (selection): *Occasional:* infusion reactions including anaphylactic shock, increased susceptibility to infection, heat flushes, hepatic dysfunction, neurologic effects (headache, dizziness, drowsiness), gastrointestinal effects (nausea, dyspepsia, diarrhea), dermatologic effects (rash, pruritus etc.). Other rare adverse effects. On re-exposure following a long treatment pause the onset of action is 3–12 days, and delayed hypersensitivity reactions may occur. Infections (e.g. tuberculosis) may be reactivated (usually within the first few weeks).

Monitoring: After each infusion patients should be monitored for at least 1–2 hours (emergency equipment!). Patients should be monitored closely throughout treatment and for up to six months thereafter for signs of infection (including tuberculosis).

Etanercept

(See Fig. 4.7 for structure)

Evaluation: Good efficacy (approximately 60% in rheumatoid arthritis) and good tolerability with long-lasting therapeutic response in some cases. The drug's effect is enhanced by combination with methotrexate. Experience is still limited. The drug is indicated only if the patient fails to respond to other SAARDs.

Mechanisms of action: Etanercept is a recombinant soluble TNF receptor (a fusion protein from the Fc region of human IgG_1 and two p75-TNF receptors). By reducing the amount of circulating TNF, it inhibits TNF-mediated inflammatory reactions.

Pharmacokinetics: Etanercept is slowly absorbed from the subcutaneous injection site. Peak plasma levels are reached after approximately 48 hours (bioavailability 76%). The elimination half-life is 70 hours. When etanercept is given twice weekly by injection, the steady-state plasma concentration is about twice as high as after a single injection. No increased plasma levels of etanercept were observed patients with acute renal or hepatic failure.

Indications: Rheumatoid arthritis in adults and children from four years who have not responded adequately to one or more SAARDs. Etanercept is contraindicated in patients with acute infection or in patients at risk of septicemia.

Onset of action: Very short (1–2 weeks, maximum three months).

Dosage: 25 mg subcutaneously twice weekly (in children ≥4 years and adults under 18 years 0.4 mg/kg up to a maximum dosage of 25 mg twice weekly). The injection site should be changed each time.

Adverse effects (selection): Similar to those observed with infliximab (notably an increased risk of activating latent infections, e.g. tuberculosis). Reactions at the injection site, though common, are usually mild and limited to the first month of treatment. Allergic reactions are rare. So far no neutralizing antibodies have been found.

Monitoring: Regular examinations for signs of infection.

3.5 References

Bombardier C, Laine L, Reicin A et al. Comparison of upper gastrointestinal toxicity of rofecoxib and naproxen in patients with rheumatoid arthritis. N Engl J Med 2000; 343: 1520–1528

Brune K, Zeilhofer HU. Antipyretic (non-narcotic) analgesics. In: Wall PD, Melzack R (eds). Textbook of Pain. Edinburgh: Churchill Livingston, 1999: 1139–1154

Chandrasekharan NV, Dai H, Roos KL, Evanson NK, Tomsik J. COX-3, a cyclooxygenase-1 variant inhibited by acetaminophen and other analgesic/antipyretic drugs: cloning, structure, and expression. Proc Natl Acad Sci USA 2002; 99: 13 926–13 931

Ferreira SH. Prostaglandins, aspirin-like drugs and analgesia. Nature 1972; 240: 200–203

FitzGerald GA, Patrono C. The coxibs, selective inhibitors of cyclooxygenase-2. N Engl J Med 2001; 345: 433–442

Flower RJ, Rothwell NJ. Lipocortin-1: cellular mechanisms and clinical relevance. Trends Pharmacol Sci 1994; 15: 71–76

Fu JY, Masferrer JL, Seibert K, Raz A, Needleman P. The induction and suppression of prostaglandin H_2 synthase (cyclooxygenase) in human monocytes. J Biol Chem 1990; 265: 16 737–16 740

Henrich WL. Nephrotoxicity of nonsteroidal antiinflammatory drugs. In: Little, Brown (eds). Disease of the Kidney. Vol. 2. 4th ed. Boston, 1988

Hinz B, Brune K. Cyclooxygenase-2 – 10 years later. J Pharmacol Exp Ther 2002; 300: 367–375

Katz WA. Pharmacology and clinical experience with tramadol in osteoarthritis. Drugs 1996; 52 (Suppl 3): 39–47

Komers R, Anderson S, Epstein M. Renal and cardiovascular effects of selective cyclooxygenase-2 inhibitors. Am J Kidney Dis 2001; 38: 1145–1157

Laine L, Harper S, Simon T et al. A randomized trial comparing the effect of rofecoxib, a cyclooxygenase 2-specific inhibitor, with that of ibuprofen on the gastroduodenal mucosa of patients with osteoarthritis. Gastroenterology 1999; 117: 776–783

Miehle W. Medikamentöse Therapie rheumatischer Erkrankungen. Stuttgart: Thieme, 2000: 33

Mizuno H, Sakamoto C, Matsuda K et al. Induction of cyclooxygenase 2 in gastric mucosal lesions and its inhibition by the specific antagonist delays healing in mice. Gastroenterology 1997; 112: 387–397

Muth-Selbach S, Tegeder I, Brune K, Geisslinger G. Acetaminophen inhibits spinal prostaglandin E_2 release after peripheral noxious stimulation. Anesthesiology 1999; 91: 231–239

Perazella MA, Tray K. Selective cyclooxygenase-2 inhibitors: a pattern of nephrotoxicity similar to traditional nonsteroidal anti-inflammatory drugs. Am J Med 2001; 111: 64–67

Pinsky PR, Hurwitz ES, Schonberger LB, Gunn WJ. Reye's syndrome and aspirin. Evidence of a dose-response effect. JAMA 1988; 260: 657–661

Riendeau D, Percival MD, Brideau C et al. Etoricoxib (MK-0663): preclinical profile and comparison with other agents that selectively inhibit cyclooxygenase-2. J Pharmacol Exp Ther 2001; 296: 558–566

Rossat J, Maillard M, Nussberger J, Brunner HR, Burnier M. Renal effects of selective cyclooxygenase-2 inhibition in normotensive salt-depleted subjects. Clin Pharmacol Ther 1999; 66: 76–84

Saxena PN, Beg MMA, Singhal KC, Ahmad M. Prostaglandin-like activity in the cerebrospinal fluid of febrile patients. Indian J Med Res 1979; 79: 495–498

Schwartz JI, Vandormael K, Malice MP et al. Comparative effects of rofecoxib, celecoxib, and naproxen on renal function in elderly subjects receiving a normal-salt diet. Clin Pharmacol Ther 2002 (im Druck)

Silverstein FE, Faich G, Goldstein JL et al. Gastrointestinal toxicity with celecoxib vs nonsteroidal anti-inflammatory drugs for osteoarthritis and rheumatoid arthritis. JAMA 2000; 284: 1247–1255

Simmons DL, Botting RM, Robertson PM, Madsen ML, Vane JR. Induction of an acetaminophen-sensitive cyclooxygenase with reduced sensitivity to nonsteroid antiinflammatory drugs. Proc Natl Acad Sci USA 1999; 96: 3275–3280

Swan SK, Rudy DW, Lasseter KC et al. Effect of cyclooxygenase-2 inhibition on renal function in elderly persons receiving a low-salt diet. A randomized, controlled trial. Ann Intern Med 2000; 133: 1–9

Vane JR. Inhibition of prostaglandin synthesis as a mechanism of action for the aspirin-like drugs. Nature 1971; 231: 232–235

Vane JR, Botting RM. Mechanism of action of anti-inflammatory drugs. Scand J Rheumatol 1996; 25 (Suppl 102): 9–21

White WB, Faich G, Whelton A et al. Comparison of thromboembolic events in patients treated with celecoxib, a cyclooxygenase-2 specific inhibitor, versus ibuprofen or diclofenac. Am J Cardiol 2002; 89: 425–430

Wolfe MM, Lichtenstein DR, Singh G. Gastrointestinal toxicity of nonsteroidal antiinflammatory drugs. N Engl J Med 1999; 340: 1888–1899

4 New and Future Therapeutic Approaches

Stefan Laufer

4.1 Introduction

Since the discovery of the first antirheumatic drug, acetylsalicylic acid, in 1899, more than 100 drugs have been introduced worldwide for the treatment of rheumatic diseases. This clearly reflects the importance of this drug group as well as the high demand for new antirheumatic drugs. Evidently there is both room for and a need for further improvements.

This chapter discusses drugs that are currently in an advanced stage of development and are expected to be marketed in the foreseeable future. It then presents a selection of research avenues that are being intensively pursued at the moment, providing a window onto promising future developments.

4.2 Drugs in advanced stages of clinical development

COX-2 inhibitors

Celecoxib and rofecoxib were the first selective inhibitors of cyclooxygenase-2 (COX-2) to reach the market. However, it soon emerged that that these drugs leave some room for improvement. Consequently, second-generation drugs of this class are already in the pipeline. It was discovered during regulatory studies that the analgesic potency of the coxibs is less than that of convention nonsteroidal anti-inflammatory drugs (NSAIDs). In several pain studies celecoxib was found to be inferior to naproxen and ibuprofen, for example [Arthritis Advisory Committee, 1998]. The lack of a parenteral dosage form is a further disadvantage for pain treatment. Optimization is also possible in terms of the COX-2 versus COX-1 selectivity ratio of this drug.

In vitro human whole blood models are considered to be most appropriate to evaluate drug selectivity [Riendeau et al., 2001]. The disparity of results from other models can be seen from meloxicam, an inhibitor whose selectivity is particularly controversial (Table 4.**1**). Almost any desired selectivity factor can be demonstrated by choosing suitable test models. The literature reports highly variable data for other NSAIDs as well (Table 4.**2**) [Dougados, 1999]. Table 4.**3** gives the inhibitory values and selectivity ratios for a number of COX-2 inhibitors and several conventional NSAIDs in the human whole blood model.

According to the literature, in June 2001 a total of 15 COX-2 inhibitors were under clinical development, namely flosulide, DuP-697, FK-3311, L-745 377, CT-3, L-752 860, JTE-522, GR-253 035, P-54, COX-189, CS-502, ABT-963, parecoxib, valdecoxib, and etoricoxib [Prous Science Database, 2001]. Here we will focus on etoricoxib, valdecoxib, and parecoxib, drugs close to the market in major countries.

Etoricoxib (MK-0663)

Etoricoxib is a time-dependent inhibitor of COX-2. With an IC_{50} of 1.1 µM for COX-2 in the human whole blood model (LPS-induced PGE_2 synthesis) and an IC_{50} value of 116 µM for COX-1 (serum TXB_2 after coagulation), the substance has a selectivity of 106, the highest selectivity of all derivatives in an advanced stage of development. It is even more selective than rofecoxib. Etoricoxib has undergone intensive preclinical testing. In animal models of acute and chronic inflammation the substance proved effective in the dosage range of 0.3 – 0.6 mg/kg (carrageenan-induced rat paw edema: ED_{50} = 0.64 mg/kg, carrageenan-induced hyperalgesia: ED_{50} = 0.34 mg/kg, adjuvant arthritis: 0.6 mg/kg). The ulcerogenic dose, i.e. the dose that induces mucosal damage in the up-

Table 4.**1** COX-2/1 selectivity of meloxicam in various in vitro test systems

Test system	IC_{50} COX-1	IC_{50} COX-2	COX-2/COX-1 ratio
Seminal vesical vs. placenta (sheep)	4×10^{-5}	6×10^{-5}	1.5
Macrophages (Guinea pig)	5.8×10^{-5}	1.9×10^{-5}	0.33
Aortic endothelial cells vs. LPS-stimulated macrophages	2.1×10^{-7}	1.7×10^{-7}	0.8
Recombinant enzymes in cells	5.8×10^{-5}	0.2×10^{-6}	0.09
Recombinant enzymes in microsomes	3.6×10^{-8}	0.4×10^{-5}	0.01

Table 4.**2** COX-2 selectivity of various NSAIDs according to the literature: variability of *in vitro* test models

NSAID	COX-2/COX-1 ratio lowest literature value	highest literature value
Diclofenac	0.067	4
Indomethacin	1.31	107.1
Piroxicam	9.4	600
Naproxen	0.6	75
Ibuprofen	0.67	53
Acetylsalicylic acid	2	167

per gastrointestinal tract, was found to be 200 mg/kg during a ten-day course of treatment in rats. This provides a large safety margin [Riendeau et al., 2001].

Unfortunately, there is a paucity of published clinical data, and it is necessary to consult congress reports, which need to be interpreted prudently. Etoricoxib was developed for the treatment of osteoarthritis, rheumatoid arthritis (chronic polyarthritis), and pain. The substance is rapidly absorbed and has an elimination half-life of 15 hours. In clinical efficacy studies etoricoxib was investigated in doses of 5–250 mg. Significant differences to placebo were observed in osteoarthritis at doses from 30 mg and in rheumatoid arthritis at doses from 90 mg. In a tooth extraction study a single dose of 120 mg was effective for 24 hours [Sorbera et al., 2001].

Valdecoxib (SC-65 872)

In the human whole blood model valdecoxib inhibits COX-2 with an IC_{50} value of 0.87 µM and COX-1 with an IC_{50} value of 26.1 µM. This gives a selectivity of 30 – a substantial improvement on celecoxib with a selectivity of 7.6. ED_{50} values of 0.03 mg/kg (adjuvant arthritis) to 10 mg/kg (rat paw edema) were found for valdecoxib in *in vivo* preclinical models of inflammation [Drug Data Report, 2000].

Clinically, the substance was developed for the treatment of osteoarthritis, rheumatoid arthritis, dysmenorrhea, and acute pain [DailyDrugNews.com, 2001 d].

As with etoricoxib, there is a dearth of published data from clinical studies. In osteoarthritis patients the substance was shown to be significantly superior to diclofenac and ibuprofen in terms of gastrointestinal tolerance [Goldstein, 2001].

Parecoxib sodium (SC-69,124 A)

This substance was developed for the treatment of acute pain by intravenous and intramuscular injection. As water-soluble prodrug, parecoxib is

Table 4.**3** Inhibitory values and selectivity ratios of various COX-2 inhibitors and some conventional NSAIDs in the human whole blood model (IC_{50} values ± SEM), in order of COX-2 selectivity

	IC_{50} COX-1 [µM]	n (Donor)	IC_{50} COX-2 [µM]	n (Donor)	COX-2 selectivity ratio IC_{50} COX-1/COX-2
Etoricoxib	116 ± 18	12	1,1 ± 0,1	26	106
Rofecoxib	18.8 ± 0.9	211	0.53 ± 0.02	614	35
Valdecoxib	26.1 ± 4.3	11	0.87 ± 0.11	14	30
Celecoxib	6.7 ± 0.9	13	0.87 ± 0.18	18	7.6
Nimesulide	4.1 ± 1.2	6	0.56 ± 0.12	6	7.3
Diclofenac	0.15 ± 0.04	10	0.05 ± 0.01	16	3.0
Etodolac	9.0 ± 2.5	3	3.7 ± 0.7	6	2.7
Meloxicam	1.4 ± 0.4	6	0.70 ± 0.28	5	2.0
Indomethacin	0.19 ± 0.02	36	0.44 ± 0.07	34	0.4
Ibuprofen	4.8 ± 3.5	5	24.3 ± 9.5	7	0.2
6-MNA	28.9 ± 5.5	3	154 ± 51	5	0.2
Piroxicam	0.76 ± 0.05	6	9.0 ± 1.3	16	0.08

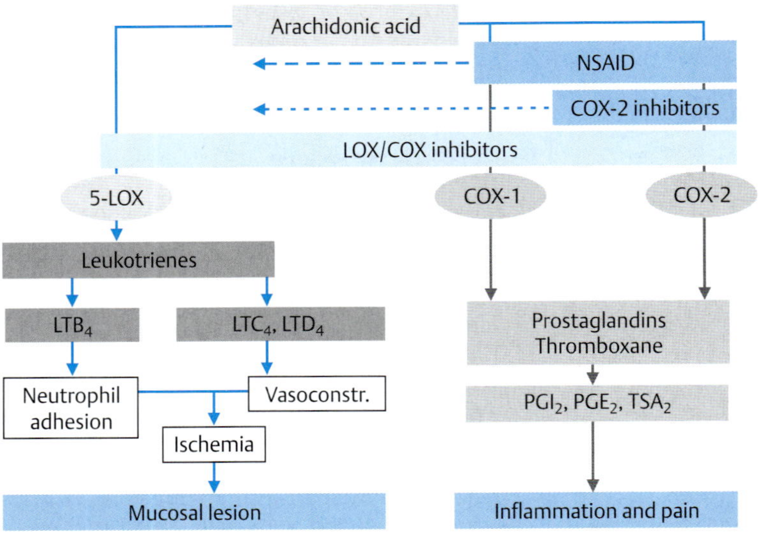

Fig. 4.**1** Shunt hypothesis of the arachidonic acid cascade after COX-1/2 inhibition.

rapidly and completely metabolized in the liver to the active form valdecoxib following parenteral administration. After intravenous administration of 1 – 200 mg the plasma half-life is five minutes. Peak plasma concentrations of valdecoxib, the active form, are reached after 0.27 – 2 h. Following intramuscular injection (1 – 40 mg) the half-life is 15 – 35 minutes and the time to peak concentration 1.1 – 3.5 h (for the active form valdecoxib).

Parecoxib is well tolerated up to a dose of 40 mg (i. m.) or 200 mg (i. v.) and does not induce irritation at the injection site. Its analgesic efficacy was investigated in clinical studies in patients undergoing tooth extraction, knee and hip surgery, and gynecologic operations. In a phase III study with 175 patients (hip replacement) 40 mg i.v. resulted in a 39% reduction of morphine use within 24 hours. Another phase III study (knee replacement) showed 40 mg parecoxib to be equivalent to 30 mg ketorolac. In several tooth extraction studies 20 – 40 mg parecoxib proved comparable to 30 – 60 mg ketorolac [DailyDrugNews.com, 2001 c; Sorbera et al., 2001]. In a study population of elderly subjects (65 – 75 years, n = 94) the substance's gastroduodenal tolerability was investigated by endoscopic examination. Given over a period of seven days, 40 mg parecoxib twice daily was significantly better tolerated than 15 mg ketorolac four times daily [Hubbard et al., 2000].

LOX/COX inhibitors

In addition to COX-2-selective inhibitors, other approaches aimed at developing gastrointestinally safe NSAIDs are being pursued. To protect the mucous membranes of the upper gastrointestinal tract a partial oxygen pressure of around 15 mm Hg is required, which can only be maintained if the microcirculation is intact [Bowen, 1981]. The improved mucosal tolerance of COX-2-selective inhibitors is due to the fact that these drugs do not suppress the synthesis of vasodilatory prostaglandins (PGE_2) by COX-1 in the stomach. Another approach is based on the so-called shunt hypothesis (Fig. 4.**1**) [Laufer, 2001].

In the presence of COX inhibition, arachidonic acid undergoes increased metabolism via the lipoxygenase (5-LOX) pathway. LTB_4 is a potent chemotactic substance and leads to enhanced adhesion of neutrophil leukocytes to the walls of postcapillary mesenteric venules. In conjunction with the vasoconstrictive activity of the cysteinyl leukotrienes LTC_4 and LTD4, microcirculation disturbances cause local ischemia and ultimately mucosal lesions. With inhibitors of COX-1/2 and 5-LOX it should be possible to circumvent this toxicity mechanism. Fig. 4.**2** shows the molecular structures of dual inhibitors in the clinical stages of development. A notable feature is the di-tertiary butyl residue, which is common to all the derivatives except licofelone (ML3000). The two enzyme systems, i.e. COX and LOX, are redox enzymes. It is therefore logical to conclude that

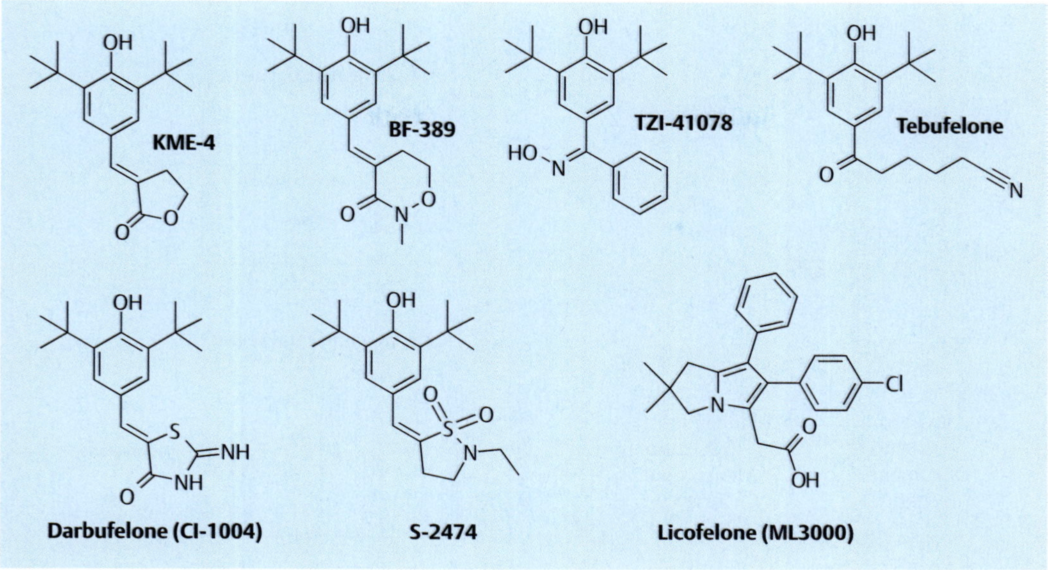

Fig. 4.**2** LOX/COX inhibitors under clinical development. Licofelone (ML3000) is a substrate analog of arachidonic acid. All other derivatives are redox inhibitors.

redoxactive structures should act as inhibitors of these enzymes. Unfortunately, this is also the crux of the problem encountered with these substances. They are not specific enough to COX and LOX; instead they interfere with redox enzymes in the liver. For this reason, except for S-2474 (a derivative that is still in the early stages of phase II development), all developments have been halted. To avoid this problem, licofelone follows a different mechanistic approach to enzyme inhibition. Both enzymes, COX-1/2 and 5-LOX, use arachidonic acid as a substrate. It should therefore be possible to develop a substrate analog to act as an inhibitor. Licofelone is such a substrate analog, which is able to simulate the conformation of arachidonic acid in the active sites of both enzymes (Fig. 4.**3**). The substance competitively inhibits COX-1, COX-2, and 5-LOX in the submicromolar concentration range (0.16–0.18 µM).

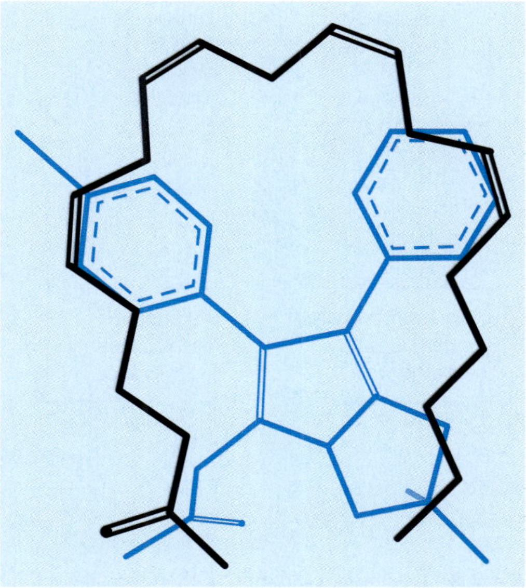

Fig. 4.**3** Conformational model of licofelone (ML3000) (blue) and arachidonic acid (black) in the active center of 5-LOX.

Licofelone has undergone intensive preclinical testing [Tries and Laufer, 2001] which validated the rationale behind LOX/COX inhibition (Fig. 4.**4**). Like conventional NSAIDs (e.g. diclofenac and indomethacin), the substance inhibits PGE_2 production in the stomach. However, with licofelone no shunt into the lipoxygenase pathway occurs. LTB_4 is not increased by licofelone as it is by diclofenac and indomethacin. Hence, significantly less leukocyte adhesion occurs at postcapillary mesenteric venules, with the result that gastric toxicity is practically absent.

This mechanism of action offers a number of advantages over COX-2 inhibitors. Because of

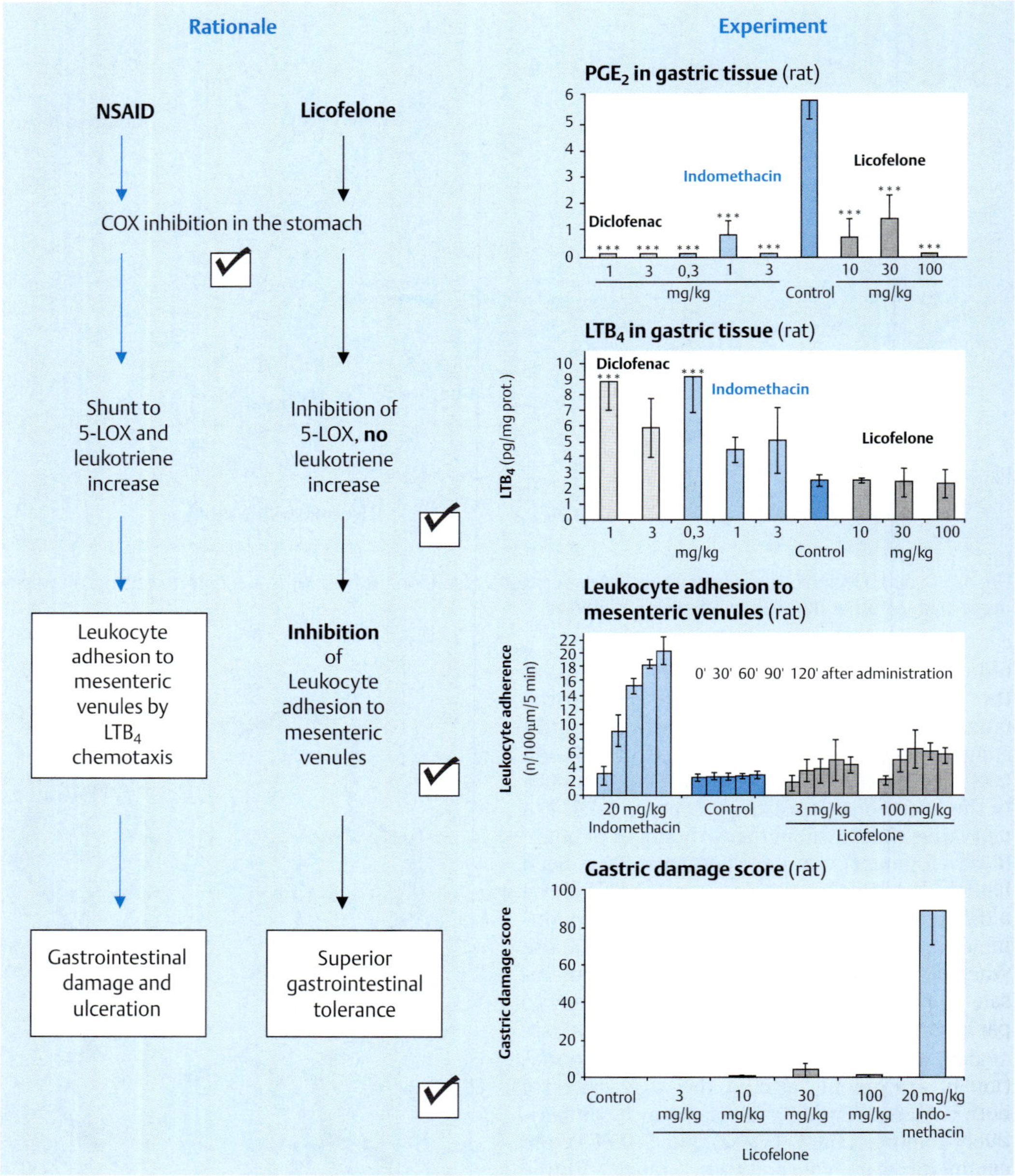

Fig. 4.**4** Preclinical validation of the rationale of inhibition of LOX/COX with licofelone.

COX-1 inhibition, the cardiovascular side effects (fluid retention, hypertension, no reduced risk of myocardial and cerebral infarction) of the COX-2 inhibitors should be absent. In addition, 5-LOX inhibition offers other pharmacodynamic options such as antiasthmatic [Abraham et al., 1997] and chondroprotective [Jovanovic et al., 2001] activity. The cysteinyl leukotrienes LTC_4/LTD_4 are potent bronchoconstrictors, and LTB_4 induces via IL-1β the activation of various matrix metalloproteinases that accelerate cartilage breakdown.

Licofelone is being developed for the treatment of osteoarthritis and is in a late stage of clinical development in Europe. Several studies from the clinical development program are pub-

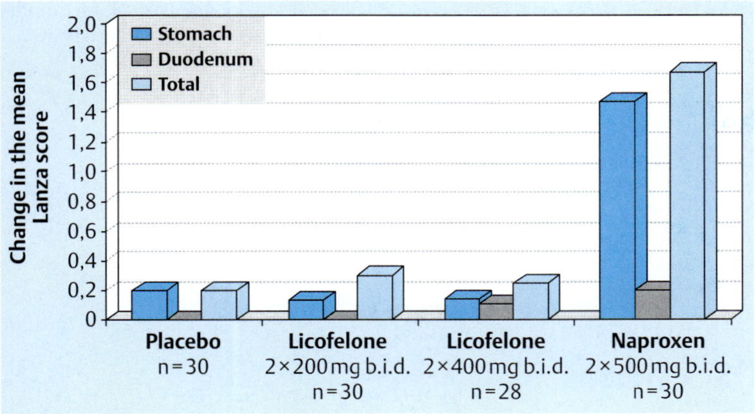

Fig. 4.**5** Endoscopic study to investigate the gastrointestinal tolerance of licofelone (118 subjects, four weeks treatment, evaluation of gastrointestinal damage by the Lanza score).

lished. In an efficacy study 404 osteoarthritic patients received 100, 200 and 400 mg licofelone b.i.d., placebo or 50 mg diclofenac t.i.d. [Reginster, 2001]. The duration of treatment in this phase I dose-finding and efficacy study was four weeks. All three licofelone doses were significantly more effective than placebo. The efficacy of both higher doses was comparable to that of diclofenac. 400 mg licofelone b.i.d. was found to be only slightly more effective than 200 mg b.i.d., so that 200 mg b.i.d. was the highest dose used in subsequent phase III studies. The adverse reaction rate with 100 mg or 200 mg licofelone b.i.d. was not higher than that observed in the placebo group, whereas, as expected, in the diclofenac group tolerance was poorer (including a bleeding gastric ulcer). Diclofenac also resulted in a significant elevation of transaminases, whereas in all the licofelone groups all laboratory safety parameters, including hepatic and renal parameters, remained unchanged.

A study with 118 female and male subjects (mean age 42 years) investigated the gastroduodenal tolerance of four weeks' treatment with 200 mg and 400 mg licofelone b.i.d. (i.e. the therapeutic dose and twice the therapeutic dose) in comparison to placebo and 500 mg naproxen b.i.d. [Reginster, 2001]. In an endoscopic follow-up examination after four weeks ulcers were found in 20% of the subjects in the naproxen group, whereas no ulcerations occurred in the other groups (Fig. 4.**5**). After completion of treatment with naproxen only 37% of the subjects had a fully intact gastric mucosa. In the three other treatment groups this was the case in approximately 90% of the subjects. Both in terms of manifest ulcerations and mucosal erosions, tolerance of licofelone in the dosages mentioned was comparable to that observed with placebo.

It can be concluded from the results of the two studies that licofelone is about as effective as diclofenac in patients with osteoarthritis, while both gastrointestinal tolerance and the systemic tolerance are significantly superior to those of conventional NSAIDs.

NO-NSAIDs (Nitro-NSAIDs)

As explained in the foregoing section, intact microcirculation is essential for good gastrointestinal tolerance. NO-NSAIDs support the microcirculation in the gastrointestinal mucosa by releasing the vasodilatory substance nitrogen monoxide (NO). This is meant to compensate for the absence of gastroprotective (vasodilating) prostaglandins resulting from COX-1 inhibition [Kulkarni et al., 2001].

Fig. 4.**6** shows derivatives that are currently under clinical development. The substances are prodrugs which are metabolically converted to the corresponding NSAID, releasing NO in the process. All the compounds follow the same chemical strategy. They consist of a known NSAID coupled via a metabolically unstable linker to an NO group. Some of the developers of these derivatives even claim an intrinsic activity of NO-NSAIDs based on inhibition of inducible NO synthase [Baydoun et al., 1995]. On the other hand, NO is known to be a proinflammatory agent. Other questions concerning potential inbalance of blood pressure regulation remain open. Vasodilating properties have been described [Adami et al., 1996]. Overall, the soundness of the concept of NO-NSAIDs has not yet been established. Clari-

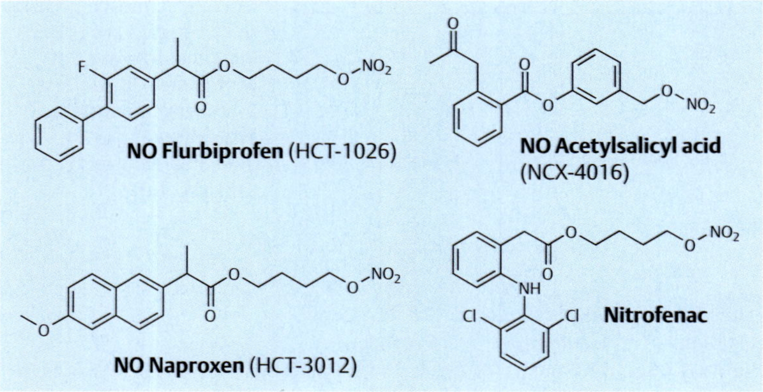

Fig. 4.**6** NO-NSAIDs under clinical development.

ty will have to await confirmatory clinical studies.

Nitrofenac

Nitrofenac is a diclofenac derivative, containing NO as nitric acid ester linked to the molecule via a 1,4-butandiole residue. Nitrofenac has been the subject of extensive preclinical testing and exhibits good activity in acute and chronic inflammation models with superior gastrointestinal tolerance compared to diclofenac [Conforti et al., 1993; Wallace et al., 1994]. Clinical data have yet to be published. Nitrofenac is believed to be in an early stage of clinical testing.

NO-naproxen (HCT-3012)

In preclinical tests NO-naproxen was also shown to have a significant effect in acute and chronic inflammation models in the rat together with good gastrointestinal tolerance [Cuzzolin et al., 1995; Drug Data Report, 1995]. Unfortunately, no clinical data are reported till now, the only thing known is that clinical pilot studies have been started [DailyDrugNews.com, 2001 a].

NO-flurbiprofen (HCT-1026)

NO-flurbiprofen is probably the NO-NSAID that has been studied in greatest detail. In addition to its anti-inflammatory properties it has also been found to inhibit osteoclast activity and to have a positive effect on irritation of the urinary bladder [Burgaud et al., 1999]. The substance was also tested topically in the form of a 1 % ointment for the treatment of acute contact urticaria [DailyDrugNews. com, 2001 b]. In a seven-day gastroscopy study 50 mg and 100 mg were compared to 100 mg flurbiprofen. Both doses were found to be better tolerated by the gastrointestinal tract than the comparator substance. Other clinical studies, including use in hyperactive bladder and osteoporosis, are under way [DailyDrugNews. com, 2000 b and 2000 d]. The results are not known.

NO-acetylsalicylic acid (NCX-4016)

Unlike the other derivatives we have discussed so far, NO-acetylsalicylic acid contains a 3-hydroxybenzyl residue as a spacer and is therefore only slowly metabolized [Cirino et al., 1997]. This is meant to compensate for the short half-life of the resulting acetylsalicylic acid. The compound exhibits good gastrointestinal tolerance and has been used in rats at doses of up to 500 mg/kg without appreciable gastric damage being observed. In an animal model the drug's antiplatelet action is comparable to that of acetylsalicylic acid [Drug Data Report 1997 a, 1997 b]. The preclinical profile of NO-acetylsalicylic acid is promising. NO-acetylsalicylic acid exhibits many pharmacodynamic characteristics of acetylsalicylic acid but with better tolerance [Al-Swayeh et al., 2000]. The compound is therefore being developed initially for the treatment of pain and inflammation and later also as an antiplatelet agent. The first clinical kinetic and tolerance studies are reported to be underway [DailyDrugNews.com, 2000 a].

Anticytokine therapy

After impressive success was achieved with etanercept and infliximab in the treatment of rheumatoid arthritis and chronic inflammatory bowel disease (Figs. 4.**7** and 4.**8**), the principle of anticy-

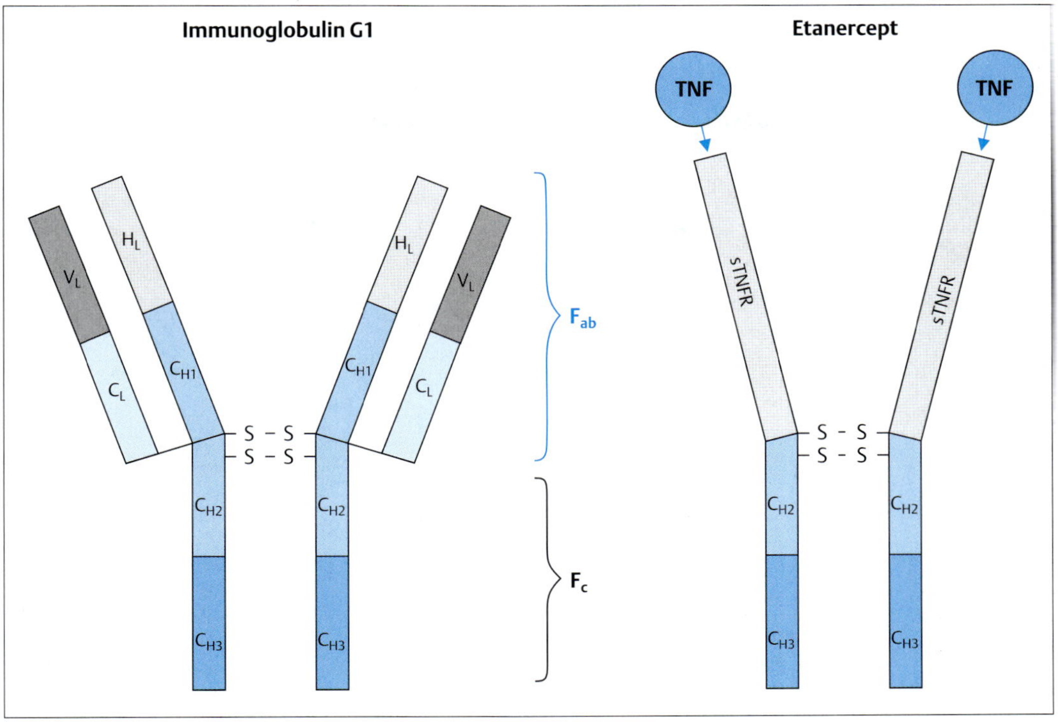

Fig. 4.**7** Etanercept is a fusion protein from the extracellular ligand-binding domain of the human 75-kDa TNF receptor (p75) and the Fc domain of human immunoglobulin G_1.

tokine therapy was regarded as clinically validated. Both drugs have been approved since 1999. Both etanercept and infliximab reduce the amount of TNF-α circulating in the blood. TNF-α and IL-1 are the most important proinflammatory cytokines. They are produced by monocytes and macrophages and act on inflammatory cells, where they induce the production of important enzymes (COX-2, MMP, iNOS, $cPLA_2$) and other factors (adhesion molecules, IL-6, chemokines) that initiate and maintain inflammation (Fig. 4.**9**).

Other drugs which are in a later stage of development or are already under regulatory review and which essentially rely on the same mechanism of action are referred to as "biologicals" in the lay press. Below we describe several representatives of this group which are in an advanced phase of clinical development for the treatment of inflammatory diseases (adalimumab, humicade and anakinra).

Adalimumab (D2E7)

Adalimumab is a recombinant 100% human monoclonal anti-hTNF-α antibody. It is a further development of infliximab, a chimeric antibody that still contains murine segments. Consequently, adalimumab should be less immunogenic, have fewer allergic side effects, and should remain longer active than its partly murine counterpart. One problem with infliximab is that efficacy wanes after just 6–12 months, as the body is likely to produce antibodies that neutralize the substance. This can be delayed by co-administering methotrexate.

Adalimumab has a high affinity for human TNF-α with a K_d value of 0.6 nM. In clinical phase I/II studies response to the treatment was observed over a period of several years [Drug Data Report, 1997 c]. However, in the confirmatory studies the substance was combined with methotrexate. 1 mg/kg twice weekly i.v. or s.c. (with 15 mg methotrexate weekly) given to 54 patients with rheumatoid arthritis resulted in a response rate (ACR 20) of 70% compared to 28% in the pla-

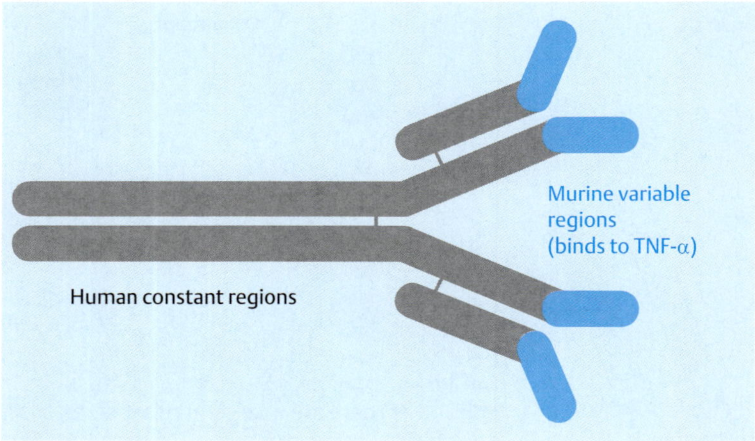

Fig. 4.**8** Infliximab is a chimeric monoclonal antibody to TNF-α. The constant region comes from human IgG_1, while the variable antigen-binding portion is of murine origin.

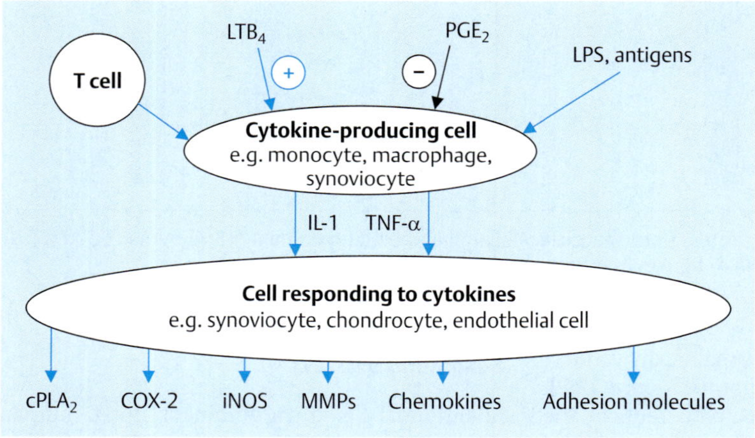

Fig. 4.**9** The proinflammatory cytokines TNF-α and IL-1 produced by monocytes and macrophages stimulate various reactive cells to synthesize enzymes that strengthen and maintain the inflammation.

cebo group. Effects were evident after just two weeks [Rau, 1999]. Further efficacy data are known from a two-year study [Breedveld, 2001]. As is the case with many drugs under development, published efficacy and tolerance data are scarce. The drug is expected to be marketed in 2003 [DailyDrugNews.com, 2001 e].

Humicade (CDP-571, Bay-10-3356)

Humicade is a recombinant humanized monoclonal IgG_4 anti-TNF-α antibody in which the complementary determining regions (CDRs) originate from murine antibody CB0010. The substance is reported to have little immunogenicity. The murine portion comprises about 5% of the molecule. Humicade has a high affinity (K_d= 0.1 nM) for human TNF-α. In a pilot study with an observation period of eight weeks in patients with Crohn's disease the Crohn's Disease Activity Index was significantly reduced two weeks after a single infusion of 5 mg/kg. The effect did not persist. In a six-month dose-finding study in the same indication the optimum dose proved to be 10 mg/kg every 12 weeks. The apparent half-life was found to be 4–5 days. Other studies confirmed the possibility of reducing steroid administration [Sorbera et al., 2000]. Humicade was also developed for the treatment of rheumatoid arthritis. To date no study results have been published.

Anakinra (rhIL-1 ra)

Anakinra is a recombinant human IL-1 receptor antagonist. It was isolated from human monocytes and cloned and expressed in *E. coli.* As shown in Fig. 4.**9**, IL-1 acts on inflammatory cells, stimulating them to express other inflammation-relevant enzymes and factors. Anakinra neutralizes circulating IL-1, resulting in anti-inflammatory effects.

The drug has so far been developed solely for the treatment of rheumatoid arthritis and is now undergoing regulatory review in the USA. Its efficacy and tolerance have been investigated in over 3000 patients [DailyDrugNews.com, 2000 c]. Anakinra, though significantly more effective than placebo, is less effective than TNF-α antibodies. Response rates (ACR 20) were only 10–15% better than with placebo. Since IL-1 and TNF-α stimulate the expression of each other, a combination of drugs directed against both cytokines would be possible. Preclinical data have confirmed the logic of this hypothesis and demonstrated synergistic effects [Feige et al., 2000]. However, if anakinra is combined with etanercept, the immunosuppressive effect is so strong that 7% of patients experience severe infection. In view of this potential adverse effect, no further combination studies were performed.

Anakinra is a reserve drug for the treatment of patients who fail to respond to DMARDs [FDA Arthritis Advisory Committee, 2001].

4.3 Drugs in the early research stage

Cytosolic phospholipase A_2 ($cPLA_2$)

The key reaction of the arachidonic acid cascade is the release of arachidonic acid from phospholipids of the cell membrane. Excessive activation of this cascade leads to increased levels of many inflammation-relevant mediators, e.g. prostaglandins, leukotrienes, PAF, and lysophospholipid (see Fig. 2.**2**). Phospholipases are therefore an interesting target for new drug developments. The main problem has been the development of a reliable *in vitro* model for screening candidate inhibitors, as there are a large number of different phospholipases in the body and it was not clear which are responsible for the intracellular release of arachidonic acid. The PLA_2 enzyme family is large and heterogeneous. Although all members of the family cleave arachidonic acid from the sn-2 position of phospholipids, their location, substrate specificity, and activation are highly variable (see Table 2.**1**).

In recent years it has become increasingly clear that the 85-kD $cPLA_{2a}$ molecule is responsible for controlling intracellular arachidonic acid release and therefore plays a key role in inflammation events. Findings in knock-out mice have lent support to this hypothesis [Lehr, 2001]. The first parent structures of selective $cPLA_{2a}$ inhibitors have been described in patents (Fig. 4.**10**). So far, however, poor oral bioavailability (low absorption rate, rapid metabolism) has hindered broad-based *in vivo* validation of this mechanism.

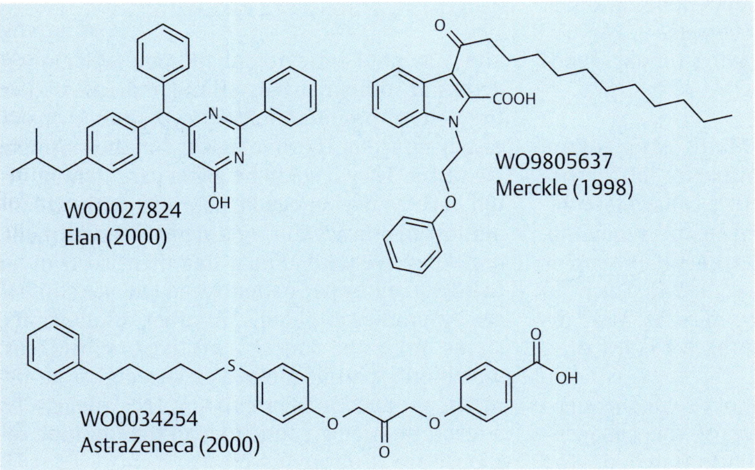

Fig. 4.**10** Molecular structures of inhibitors of $cPLA_2$.

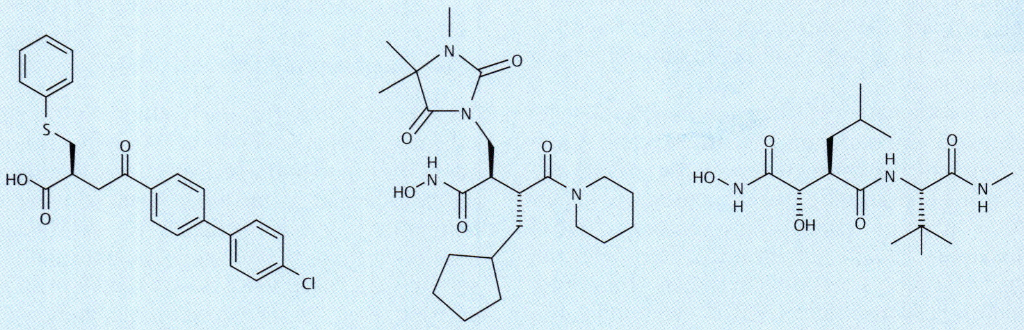

Tanomastat **Cipemastat** **Marimastat**

Fig. 4.**11** Matrix metalloproteinase inhibitors under clinical development.

Matrix metalloproteinase inhibitors

Matrix metalloproteinases (MMPs) form a family of zinc-containing enzymes that break down all major components of the extracellular matrix. Their expression is strictly regulated by pro- and anti-inflammatory cytokines and growth factors. MMPs are often secreted as inactive proenzymes and are activated by removal of a propeptide region. Once activated, they can only be inhibited by stochiometric amounts of so-called tissue inhibitors [Matrisian, 1990; Woessner, 1991].

A number of diseases, e.g. arthritis, cancer, and multiple sclerosis, are associated with overexpression or overactivation of MMPs. MMPs are essentially involved in three phases of cancer progression:

- Primary tumor growth and invasion of healthy tissue.
- Metastasis, detachment, and penetration of tumor cells through blood vessels.
- Vascularization of the growing tumor, angiogenesis.

In rheumatic diseases some MMPs (stromelysin, PMN collagenase) are responsible for intra-articular cartilage degradation. High collagenase activity has been demonstrated in the synovium, and PMN collagenase is overexpressed in synovial cells (mRNA) [Brown et al., 1994]. Since no causal therapies exist for either disease, MMP inhibition is an interesting approach to new drug development.

The first-generation inhibitors were oligopeptides based on the sequence of the collagen-cleaving site. Later work concentrated on the zinc ion, which is essential for the enzymatic activity of MMPs. Hydroxamic acids and thioamides structurally dominate this class of inhibitors. More recent developments have been characterized by *de novo* design based on crystal structures [Beckett et al., 1996]. A number of derivates are under clinical development for the treatment of patients with neoplastic disease, rheumatoid arthritis, and osteoarthritis. Most advanced are studies with marimastat, cipemastat and tanomastat, which are undergoing clinical phase III testing (Fig. 4.**11**). These developments have recently been overshadowed by suspicions that these compounds may be potentially carcinogenic. To various extents many MMP inhibitors inhibit the enzyme caspase-3, which is thought to play an important role in apoptosis. The search for new selective inhibitors has begun anew.

Inhibitors of cytokine release

The success of anticytokine therapy with etanercept and infliximab has stimulated research in the field of proinflammatory cytokines. A major disadvantage of the "biologicals" is their protein character. They have to be given parenterally, often have an immunogenic potential with attendant loss of efficacy during progressive treatment, are expensive with annual treatment costs of up to 20,000 euros per patient/year, and are still beset by product problems. Another disadvantage stems from the kinetics of these substances, which only permit a more or less digital all-or-nothing reduction of circulating TNF-α levels. As a result physiologic functions in the immune response are also suppressed.

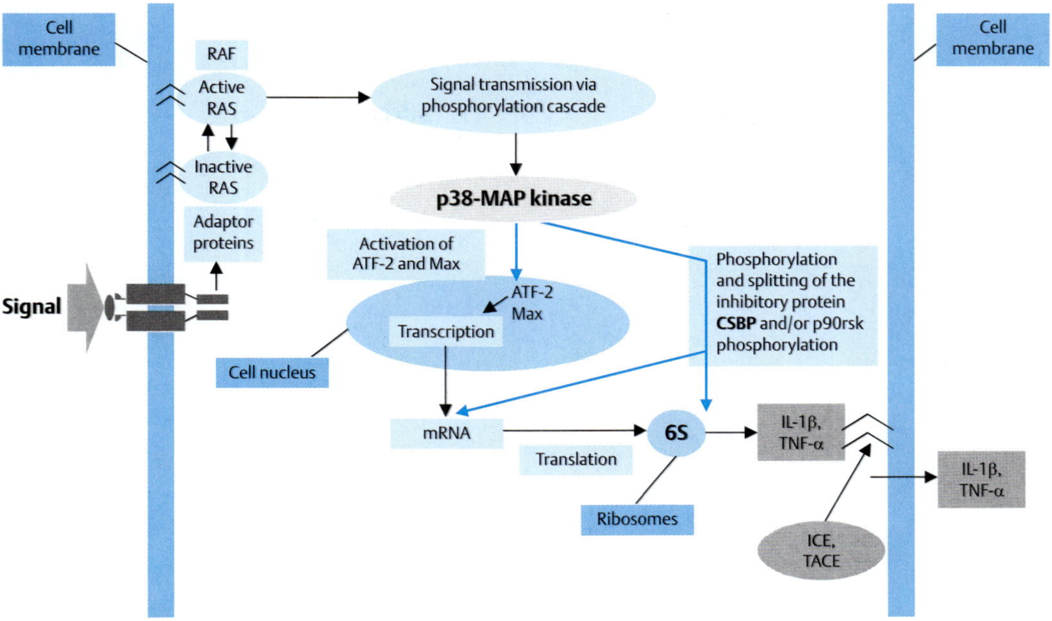

Fig. 4.**12** p-38-MAP kinase regulates the production of IL-1β and TNF-α at the transcription and translation levels.

There is therefore a demand for small molecules that avoid the disadvantages typical of peptides. Initial endeavors have concentrated on the enzymes that release IL-1β and TNF-α from their proforms (interleukin-converting enzymes, ICE, or caspase 1; TNF-α-converting enzymes, TACE). One problem that has been encountered is that pro-TNF-α is specifically split not only by TACE but also by many MMPs, whose substrate specificity is low. Selective ICE inhibitors have not proved very effective, raising the suspicion that IL-1 inhibition alone does not constitute an adequate anti-inflammatory principle.

Another approach aims to disrupt the intracellular signal transduction of cytokines. The key enzyme here is p38-MAP kinase (p38 mitogen-activated protein kinase), which was only discovered a few years ago [Lee et al., 1999]. This enzyme regulates the production of TNF-α and IL-1β at the transcription and translation levels (Fig. 4.**12**) by phosphorylating transcription factor ATF-2, which is responsible for the production of the mRNAs coding for IL-1β and TNF-α [Foster et al., 2000]. In addition, the enzyme controls translation by phosphorylating an mRNA suppressor protein (cytokine binding protein) and at the ribosomal level through interaction with p90 rsk/S6.

The pharmacologic quest for inhibitors of cytokine release began with the discovery of the prototype SKF 86 002 (Fig. 4.**13**), which was retrospectively characterized as a p38 inhibitor. This nearly 20-year-old substance attracted attention in animal experiments because of its anti-inflammatory activity, though the mode of action was unclear at the time. Inhibitors of p38-MAP kinase have been shown to be effective in preclinical tests. They reduce both TNF-α and IL-1β in the bloodstream in a dose-independent manner and synergistically inhibit the proinflammatory effect of both cytokines. In addition, several derivatives have been extensively tested in animal experiments, which have validated the underlying rationale [Badger et al., 2000]. A still unmet challenge is to achieve selectivity in space. Some 2500 kinases occur within the cell, and the object is to inhibit just one of them. The problem appears solvable, since p38-MAP kinase differs slightly from other kinases at its active site. This hope has been underpinned by *in vitro* studies with known inhibitors [Wilson et al., 1997]. Early clinical studies foundered on interactions between drug candidates and CYP-450 enzyme systems in the liver. Thus, the search for even more selective inhibitors continues.

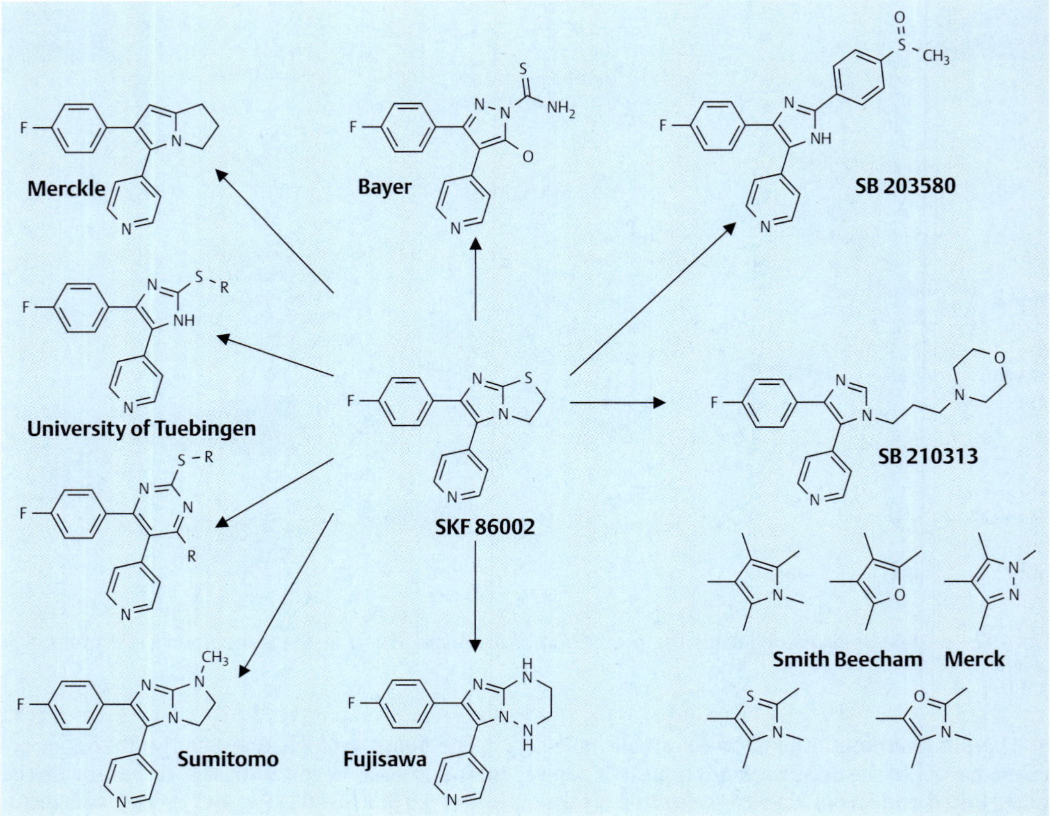

Fig. 4.**13** Molecular structures of inhibitors of p38-MAP kinase.

Gene therapy

Gene therapy based on the transfer of genetic material to somatic cells, the aim being to increase the production of specific therapeutically active proteins or reduce the biosynthesis of other pathobiochemically relevant proteins.

Early preclinical lines of research impressively demonstrated the role of various structures in the inflammatory process. These include, to mention just a few examples, IL-1Ra, IL-4, IL-10, IL-12 p40, sTNFR, NF-κB/IKK regulation, and Fas-induced apoptosis [Tsokos, 2002 a].

Theoretical considerations concerning the use of gene therapy for the treatment of inflammatory diseases (e.g. arthritis) go back more than ten years old. Most of these approaches concentrated on local gene therapy, i.e. the introduction of therapeutic genes into the synovial membrane of arthritic joints, for example. Adenovirus vectors proved suitable for this purpose in preclinical *in vivo* tests. In early studies with humans, however, difficulties were encountered in the form of inflammatory reactions triggered by adenoviral infections. For this reason *ex vivo* methods have been favored, as they do not have to contend with inflammatory reactions and are also safe, since no transducing material finds its way directly into the body. It is also possible to examine genetically modified cells in detail before they are reimplanted. The following describes the development of a specific gene therapy protocol.

The first step in the development of gene therapy strategies is to identify and validate a therapeutic target. The role of cytokines in rheumatoid arthritis has been well studied, and IL-1Ra appears to be an interesting protein whose overexpression in the synovium is believed to have a therapeutic effect.

Preclinical tests were conducted in rabbits. Biopsies of the knee joint were removed and synovial cell cultures prepared from them. The cDNA which codes for the entire human IL-1Ra was cloned in a Moloney-based retrovirus. The MFG-IRAP vector thus obtained was used to infect the synovial cell cultures. Autologously transduced cells were reimplanted into the knee joint. IL-1Ra expression was monitored for a period of six weeks. In addition, the IL-1β concentration in the synovial fluid fell, possibly as a result of inhibition of autocrine regulatory mechanisms.

Following intensive preclinical investigations that included intravenous administration (regarded as the worst case), the way was open for initial clinical phase I studies. For safety reasons the genetically modified cells were intra-articularly injected a week before elective joint replacement. Patients in this study were postmenopausal women (n = 9) with end-stage rheumatoid arthritis of the fingers who were about to undergo replacement of a metacarpophalangeal joint (2–5) and who had previously undergone surgery on another joint. During the first operation synovial biopsies were removed and autologous cell cultures were prepared. One half of the culture was transduced with MFG-IRAP, while the other half served as the control. Following extensive safety tests for endotoxins, mycoplasmas, bacteria, fungi, and replicable viruses, the cells were injected intra-articularly. Injection of non-transduced cells into other affected joints served as a control. A week later the joints were replaced. Synovial samples collected at operation were tested for gene expression by means of RT-PCR. In addition IL-1Ra in culture was assayed with an ELISA method.

Final analysis of the study is still ongoing. However, preliminary data show that there were no safety problems and that intra-articular gene transfer did in fact take place [Tsokos, 2002 b].

Acceptance of gene therapy in the therapeutic repertoire is certainly still a long way off. But the first steps have been taken and preclinical work on numerous other approaches is progressing.

4.4 References

Abraham WM, Laufer S, Tries S. The effects of ML 3000 on antigen-induced responses in sheep. Pulm Pharm Ther 1997; 10: 167–173

Adami A, Cuzzolin L, Minuz P et al. Vasodilating properties of a new non-steroidal anti-inflammatory drug, nitrofluorbiprofen, on rat aortic rings. Pharmacol Res 1996; 33: 239–244

Al-Swayeh OA, Clifford, RH, del Soldato P, Moore PK. A comparison of the anti-inflammatory and anti-nociceptive activity of nitroaspirin and aspirin. Br J Pharmacol 2000; 129: 343–350

Arthritis Advisory Committee, 1.12.1998, www.fda.-gov/search.html

Badger AM, Griswold DE, Kapadia R et al. Disease-modifying activity of SB 242 235, a selective inhibitor of p38 mitogen-activated protein kinase, in rat adjuvant-induced arthritis. Arthritis Rheum 2000; 43: 175–183

Baydoun AR et al. Elevation of cGMP in human endothelial cells by fluorbiprofen-nitroxybutylester, novel nonsteroidal anti-inflammatory drug with reduced ulcerogenic activity in vivo. Br J Pharmacol 1995; 114 (Suppl): Abstract 71 P

Beckett RP, Davidson AH, Drummond AH, Huxley P, Whittaker M. Recent advances in matrix metalloproteinase inhibitor research. Drug Discovery Today 1996; 1: 16–26

Bowen JC. In: Harmon JW (ed). Basic Mechanisms of Gastrointestinal Mucosal Cell Injury and Protection Baltimore: Williams & Wilkins, 1981: 67 ff

Breedveld FC. EULAR-Congress 13. –16.6.2001, Prag Abstract OP0062

Brown FK, Brown PJ, Bickett DM et al. Matrix metalloproteinase inhibitors containing a (carboxyalkyl) amino zinc ligand: modification of the P1 and P2 residues. J Med Chem 1994; 37: 674–688

Burgaud JL, Benedini F, Robinson EM, Del Soldato P. HCT-1026. Treatment of septic shock treatment of urinary incontinence treatment of osteoporosis nitric oxide donor. Drugs Future 1999; 24: 858–861

Cirino G, Calignano A, Sannicolo F et al. NCX-4016 Drugs Future 1997: 22: 1231–1233

Conforti A, Donini M, Brocco G et al. Acute anti-inflammatory activity and gastrointestinal tolerability of diclofenac and nitrofenac. Agents Actions 1993; 40 176–180

Cuzzolin L, Conforti A, Adami A et al. Anti-inflammatory potency and gastrointestinal toxicity of a new compound, nitronaproxen. Pharmacol Res 1995 31: 61–65

DailyDrugNews.com 27.1.2000 (2000 a)

DailyDrugNews.com 15.5.2000 (2000 b)

DailyDrugNews.com 17.11.2000 (2000 c)

DailyDrugNews.com 29.11.2000 (2000 d)

DailyDrugNews.com 24.1.2001 (2001 a)

DailyDrugNews.com 20.4.2001 (2001 b)

DailyDrugNews.com 24.4.2001 (2001 c)

DailyDrugNews.com 7.5.2001 (2001 d)

DailyDrugNews.com 22.5.2001 (2001 e)

Dougados M. 4th World Congress on Inflammation, Paris 27. –30.6.1999. Satellite Symposium: The role of COX-2 in Health and Disease

Drug Data Report 1995; 17 (8): 753

Drug Data Report 1997 a; 19 (3): 241

Drug Data Report 1997 b; 19 (8): 738

Drug Data Report 1997 c; 19 (11): 991

Drug Data Report 2000; 22 (5): 454

FDA Arthritis Advisory Commitee. FDA panel recommends Amgen's Kineret in rheumatoid arthritis. SCRIP No 2671, 22.8.2001, p. 20
Feige U, Hu YL, Gasser J et al. Anti-interleukin-1 and anti-tumor necrosis factor-alpha synergistically inhibit adjuvant arthritis in Lewis rats. Cell Mol Life Sci 2000; 57: 1457 - 1470
Foster ML, Halley F, Souness JE. Potential of p38 inhibitors in the treatment of rheumatoid arthritis. Drug News Perspect 2000; 13: 488 - 497
Goldstein JL. Digestive Disease Week, 20. - 23. Mai 2001, Atlanta, USA, Abstract 3032
Hubbard RC, Kuss ME, LeComte DL et al. An endoscopic study of the gastroduodenal effects of SC-69,124 A, a parenteral COX-2-specific inhibitor, in the elderly. Gastroenterology 2000; 118 (Suppl 2): A250
Jovanovic DV, Fernandes JC, Martel-Pelletier J et al. In vivo dual inhibition of cyclooxygenase and lipoxygenase by ML-3000 reduces the progression of experimental osteoarthritis: suppression of collagenase 1 and interleukin-1 beta synthesis. Arthritis Rheum 2001; 44: 2320 - 2330
Kulkarni SK, Jain NK, Singh A. Nitric oxide-releasing NSAIDs: A new dimension in nonsteroidal antiinflammatory drugs. Drugs Future 2001; 26: 485 - 489
Laufer S. Discovery and development of ML3000. Inflammopharmacology 2001; 9: 101 - 112
Lee JC, Kassis S, Kumar S, Badger A, Adams JL. p38 mitogen-activated protein kinase inhibitors - mechanisms and therapeutic potentials. Pharmacol Ther 1999; 82: 389 - 397
Lehr M. Phospholipase A_2 inhibitors in inflammation. Expert Opin Ther Patents 2001; 11: 1123 - 1136
Matrisian LM. Metalloproteinases and their inhibitors in matrix remodeling. Trends Genet 1990; 6: 121 - 125
Prous Science Database, 2001, Barcelona, Spain
Rau R. EULAR-Congress, 6. - 11. Juni 1999, Glasgow, Abstract 907
Reginster JY. ML3000 - Recent Clinical Trials. Eular Congress, Satellite Symposium, 15.6.2001, Prag
Riendeau D, Percival MD, Brideau CJ et al. Etoricoxib (MK-0663): preclinical profile and comparison with other agents that selectively inhibit cyclooxygenase-2. Pharm Exp Ther 2001; 296: 558 - 566
Sorbera LA, Castaner RM, Silvestre J, Castaner J. Etoricoxib: Analgesic drug, antiarthritic, cyclooxygenase-2 inhibitor. Drugs Future 2001; 26: 346 - 353
Sorbera LA, Leeson PA, Castaner J, Castaner RM. Valdecoxib and Parecoxib sodium. Analgesic, antiarthritic, cyclooxygenase-2 inhibitor. Drugs Future 2001; 26: 133 - 140
Sorbera LA, Martin L, Leeson PA. CDP-571. Treatment of IBD, anti-TNF-α MAb. Drugs Future 2000; 25: 669 - 673
Tries S, Laufer S. The pharmacological profile of ML3000: A new pyrrolizine derivative inhibiting the enzymes cyclo-oxygenase and 5-lipoxygenase. Inflammopharmacology 2001; 9: 113 - 124
Tsokos GC (ed). Modern Therapeutics in Rheumatic Diseases. Totowa: Humana Press, 2002 a: 505 - 581
Tsokos GC (ed). Modern Therapeutics in Rheumatic Diseases. Totowa: Humana Press, 2002 b: 583 - 591
Wallace JL, Reuter B, Cicala C et al. A diclofenac derivative without ulcerogenic properties. Eur J Pharmacol 1994; 257: 249 - 255
Wilson KP, McCaffrey PG, Hsiao K et al. The structural basis for the specificity of pyridinylimidazole inhibitors of p38 MAP kinase. Chem Biol 1997; 4: 423 - 431
Woessner JF. Matrix metalloproteinases and their inhibitors in connective tissue remodeling. FASEB J 1991; 5: 2145 - 2154

5 Clinical Indications for Drug Therapy

Kay Brune

5.1 Treatment goals

For most inflammatory rheumatic diseases no causal therapy is available. To a certain extent infectious arthritis and reactive arthritis are exceptions, where the objective is to eradicate the pathogen or causative agents. The aim of treatment in most cases is therefore to maintain or improve the quality of life of patients with rheumatic disease. Therapeutic efforts focus on the following measures:

1. Relief of pain.
2. Depending on the clinical picture, suppression of the inflammatory reaction in order to minimize connective-tissue destruction and maintain the patient's activity and joint function.
3. Suppression of an excessive connective-tissue reaction (e.g. pannus formation in rheumatoid arthritis) in order to prevent mutilating joint destruction.

Table 5.**1** gives an overview of the current treatment methods for rheumatic diseases. The following sections discuss in some detail the most important clinical pictures (the selection inescapably being somewhat arbitrary).

5.2 Rheumatoid arthritis

Clinical features. This chronic inflammatory joint disease (synonym: chronic polyarthritis) affects around 1% of the population. The condition is two to three times more common in women than in men with the peak incidence occurring between the ages of 40 and 70. The clinical picture can vary considerably. However, typical manifestations include symmetrical involvement of several large and small joints with painful swelling and generalized symptoms such as morning stiffness, lack of energy, and weight loss. The clinical course is also extremely variable, ranging from mild self-limiting arthritis to rapidly progressive joint destruction and inflammatory multiple-organ involvement associated with high morbidity and mortality rates.

Diagnosis and differential diagnosis. Because of its gradual onset, several months may elapse before an unambiguous diagnosis is made. The diagnostic criteria formulated by the American Rheumatism Association (ARA) have proved useful in identifying the disease (Table 5.**2**). According to this scheme, the diagnosis is deemed to be reliable if at least four of the seven criteria are met; the findings for the first four criteria must have persisted for at least six weeks.

However, it should be noted that the ARA criteria were not developed for bedside diagnosis by rather for the classification of large numbers of patients in connection with epidemiologic, clinical, and follow-up studies. Hence, even if the criteria do not apply in an individual case, this does not necessarily rule out the diagnosis of rheumatoid arthritis, especially in the early stages. However, arthralgia alone without objective joint findings is not in itself sufficient for the suspected diagnosis of rheumatoid arthritis. An early sign of rheumatoid arthritis is the gradual onset of persistent symmetrical involvement of several joints (especially those typical of the disease), a moderately increased ESR (40–60 mg/h), and typical radiologic findings (bone calcification near the joint, destruction of boundary lamellae).

Rheumatoid arthritis must be distinguished above all from diseases accompanied by chronic polyarticular inflammation. These include, notably, collagen diseases and seronegative spondylarthritides. Whereas the former are usually identified by characteristic skin lesions, a typical organ involvement pattern, and specific antibodies, spondylarthritides often pose a daunting differential diagnostic challenge, especially when peripheral joints are affected. They often take a chronic, joint-destructive course with synovial hypertrophy and histologic changes similar to those seen in rheumatoid arthritis. Peripheral joint involvement tends to be asymmetrical, and usually the large joints and (except in psoriatic arthritis) the lower extremities are affected. In psoriatic arthritis the distal phalangeal joints are mainly affected, especially in conjunction with disease of the fingernails of the affected digits. Reiter's syndrome, ankylosing spondylitis, and less consistently also enteropathic arthritis are usually accompanied by marked reddening and swelling of individual metatarsophalangeal and interphalangeal joints. This distribution is unusual for rheumatoid arthritis. Important distinguishing features of seronegative spondylarthritis include sacroiliitis, thoracic and lumbar spondylitis, and often iridocyclitis. The association of these diseases with the HLA-B27 haplotype can also be used for differential diagnosis.

Drug therapy. Because of the few reliable prognostic indicators available, close monitoring of disease activity, treatment response, and potential side-effects of the drugs used are essential

Table 5.1 Treatment options for rheumatic diseases (modified from Brune et al., 2001)

Disease	(Para)causal therapy	Symptomatic therapy: Primary therapy	Symptomatic therapy: Supportive therapy
Chronic polyarthritis			
▪ Rheumatoid arthritis (RA)	ø	SAARDs/"biologicals"[1], glucocorticoids, NSAIDs	Physiotherapy/ergotherapy, training, ortheses, synoviortheses, aids, surgical measures
▪ Juvenile chronic arthritis	ø	SAARDs, glucocorticoids, NSAIDs	As in RA
Seronegative spondylarthritides/ spondylarthropathies			
▪ Ankylosing spondylitis	ø	NSAIDs, glucocorticoids, SAARDs[2]	Physiotherapy, training, possibly surgical measures
▪ Psoriatic arthritis	ø	NSAIDs, glucocorticoids, SAARDs[3]	physiotherapy, thalassotherapy, possibly surgical measures
Reactive arthritides			
▪ Rheumatic fever	Antibiotic	NSAIDs, glucocorticoids [4]	Bedrest (+ benzodiazepines)
▪ Reiter's syndrome	ø	NSAIDs ± analgesics, rarely glucocorticoids, SAARDs in chronic cases	Bedrest, passive physiotherapy
▪ Lyme arthritis	Antibiotic	NSAIDs, glucocorticoids p. o, i. a.[5]	Cryotherapy, effusion puncture, possibly synovectomy
▪ Arthritis associated with chronic intestinal diseases	ø	NSAIDs, glucocorticoids, sulfasalazine, MTX	(MTX esp. in the case of ocular manifestation)
Infectious arthritides			
▪ Bacterial	Antibiotic[6]	NSAIDs	Joint drainage, possibly surgical débridement, synovectomy, cryotherapy
Collagen diseases/vasculitides			
▪ Systemic lupus erythematosus	ø	NSAIDs, glucocorticoids, (hydroxy) chloroquine, azathioprine, cyclophosphamide	Adjuvant therapy depending on organ manifestation
▪ Progressive systemic sclerosis (scleroderma)	ø	NSAIDs, glucocorticoids[7], vasodilators, immunosuppressants, D-penicillamine	Physiotherapy, adjuvant therapy depending on organ manifestation
▪ Sjögren's syndrome	ø	NSAIDs, (hydroxy)chloroquine	Artificial tears, avoidance of dry skin and mucous membranes
		Primary therapy	Supportive therapy

continuation next page

Table 5.1 Treatment options for rheumatic diseases (modified from Brune et al., 2001) *(continuation)*

Disease	(Para)causal therapy	Symptomatic therapy: Primary therapy	Symptomatic therapy: Supportive therapy
■ Polymyositis and dermatomyositis	ø	Glucocorticoids, MTX, cyclosporin, immune globulins, cyclophosphamide	Physiotherapy
■ Polyarteritis nodosa	ø	**Nonvirus-associated**: Glucocorticoids, immunosuppressants; **Virus-associated**: Immunosuppressants combination therapy, plasmapheresis, antiviral therapy	General infection prophylaxis
Metabolic diseases with joint symptoms			
■ Gout	ø	NSAIDs/colchicine, glucocorticoids p. o/i. a., uricosurics, uricostatics	Local cold application, avoidance of triggering factors
■ Chondrocalcinosis	ø	NSAIDs, glucocorticoids i. a.	Effusion puncture, cryotherapy, physiotherapy
■ Ochronosis	ø	NSAIDs	
■ Storage diseases, e.g. hemochromatosis	Bloodletting	NSAIDs	
Soft-tissue rheumatism			
■ Fibromyalgia	ø	Physiotherapy, amitriptyline, NSAIDs, muscle relaxants, local anesthetics	Psychotherapy, relaxation therapy
■ Insertion tendopathies	ø	NSAIDs, glucocorticoids [8]	Physiotherapy
Degenerative joint diseases (osteoarthritides)			
■ Primary osteoarthritis			
– Active	ø	Paracetamol/coxibs, NSAIDs[9], glucocorticoids	Physiotherapy etc.
– Latent	ø [10]	–	Physiotherapy, load avoidance
■ Secondary osteoarthritides			
– Functional disturbance of the musculoskeletal system	Surgery	NSAIDs	Physiotherapy
– Metabolic joint degeneration	Specific therapy	NSAIDs	Physiotherapy, surgery

Table 5.**2** 1987 revised criteria of the American Rheumatism Association (ARA) for the diagnosis of rheumatoid arthritis [after Arnett et al., 1988]

1. **Morning stiffness** in and around the joints, lasting at least one hour before maximal improvement.
2. **At least three joint areas** have soft-tissue swelling and fluid (not bony overgrowth alone) observed by a physician. The 14 possible joint areas are right or left proximal interphalangeal (PIP) joints, metacarpophalangeal (MCP) joints, wrist, elbow, knee, ankle, and metatarsophalangeal (MPT) joints.
3. At least one area swollen (as defined above) in a **wrist, MCP, or PIP joint**.
4. Simultaneous involvement of the same joint areas (see 2 above) **on both sides of the body** (bilateral involvement of PIPs, MCPs, or MTPs is acceptable without absolute symmetry).
5. **Subcutaneous nodules** over bony prominences or extensor surfaces or in juxta-articular regions observed by a physician.
6. Demonstration of **abnormal amounts of serum rheumatoid factor** by any method for which the result has been positive in < 5 % of normal control subjects.
7. **Radiographic changes** typical of rheumatoid arthritis on posteroanterior hand and wrist radiographs, which must include erosions or unequivocal bony decalcification localized to or most marked adjacent to the involved joints (osteoarthritis changes alone do not qualify).

for effective long-term treatment of rheumatoid arthritis.

The course of the disease is usually steadily progressive with intermittent acute episodes and requires lifelong complex therapy (Fig. 5.**1**). In the interest of achieving a good therapeutic response and slowing the disease progression early treatment is of key importance.

- Until the diagnosis has been confirmed, **NSAIDs** for pain relief and suppression of inflammation are given in addition to physiotherapy. Glucocorticoids are rarely used.

*Key to Table 5.**1***

MTX	Methotrexate
NSAIDs	Nonsteroidal anti-inflammatory drugs

[1] Chloroquine, gold preparations i. m., D-penicillamine, sulfasalazine, methotrexate, cyclosporin A, leflunomide, azathioprine; cyclophosphamide (combination regimens or TNF-antagonists in refractory patients)
[2] Only in peripheral joint involvement
[3] Only in progressive oligo- or polyarticular cases
[4] Only if cardiac involvement is suspected
[5] Only after antibiotic therapy, as otherwise resistance to treatment could develop
[6] According to microbial resistance tests
[7] Only in the early edematous stage of the disease and in NSAID-resistant arthritis
[8] Local infiltration
[9] Treatment for over a week is often superfluous and ineffective
[10] Efficacy of the so-called chondroprotectants and chondrotrophic drugs (glucosamine, hyaluronic acid, etc.) has not been scientifically substantiated.

- Once the diagnosis has been confirmed, systemic **combination drug therapy** should be initiated. This should include a **slow-acting antirheumatic drug** (SAARD). An **NSAID** – in cases of high disease activity an **oral glucocorticoid** (e.g. ≤ 30 mg prednisolone equivalent daily) is given instead of or in addition – serves to bridge the time until the SAARD takes effect. In elderly patients or in patients with a history of ulcers, the NSAID can be replaced by a combination of **acetaminophen and a corticosteroid.** The choice of the SAARD depends on the disease activity. Antimalarial drugs, auranofin, subreum, and pyritinol are thought to be less effective. Treatment with oral methotrexate is usually tolerated longest by patients and is now regarded by many experts as the SAARD of first choice.
- If the patient responds to the basic therapy, the glucocorticoid can be reduced or gradually withdrawn; the patient continues to take the NSAID as required or in a reduced dosage. The SAARD should be continued if remission persists, possibly in a reduced dosage.
- If complete remission is not achieved, it is advisable to proceed as follows:
  - **Local therapeutic methods** should first be exhausted (intra-articular corticosteroids, synoviortheses, synovectomy).
  - **Intensification of the drug treatment** should then be considered, e.g. a three-day regimen of high-dose intravenous corticosteroid shock therapy followed by a transi-

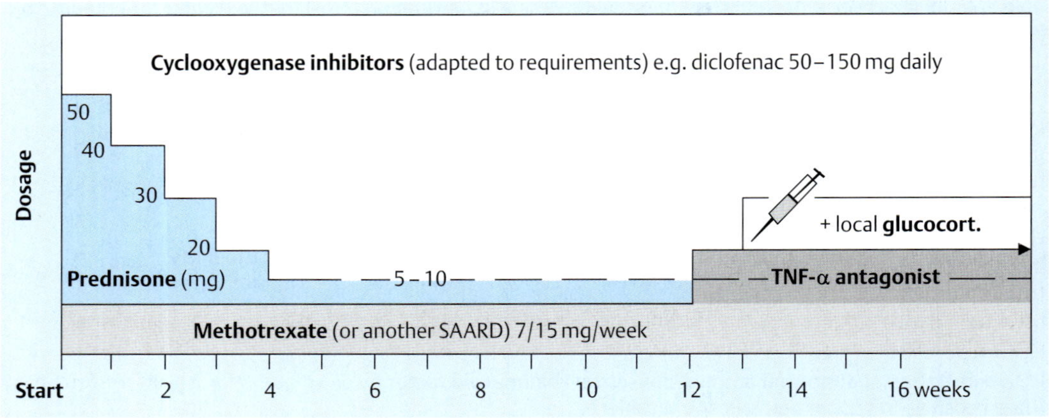

Fig. 5.**1** Treatment schedule for rheumatoid arthritis. If **two** different SAARDs do not bring about remission, treatment with TNF-α antagonists may be initiated.

tion to low-dose corticosteroid therapy, escalation of the SAARD dose (in the case of methotrexate also switching from oral to parenteral therapy with 15 to 30 mg i.v. weekly), changing the SAARD or adding another SAARD. Suitable combination partners for methotrexate are sulfasalazine + hydroxychloroquine.

- If the patient's response to the triple combination of methotrexate + sulfasalazine/hydroxychloroquine remains unsatisfactory, sulfasalazine/hydroxychloroquine can be replaced by **leflunomide.**
- If this regimen still fails to lead to remission, **etanercept,** later possibly **infliximab,** can be combined with methotrexate in place of leflunomide.

- If an inflammatory episode occurs during successful basic therapy, the patient's compliance should be checked. If compliance is ensured, the same considerations apply as when the initial SAARD proves unsatisfactory (see previous section), taking into consideration not only the disease course but also the radiologic progression. In addition, the glucocorticoid dose can be temporarily increased.

5.3 Juvenile chronic arthritis

Clinical features. The term juvenile chronic arthritis (JCA) encompasses various forms of chronic arthritis appearing in childhood or early adolescence (before the age of 16). Five forms are distinguished:

1. Polyarthritis with a systemic onset (Chauffard-Still syndrome). Onset is usually before the age of six, and girls and boys are affected almost equally. It is characterized by symmetric joint involvement, intermittent fever episodes, and severe involvement of some internal organs (hepatomegaly, splenomegaly, pericarditis, pleurisy, pneumonitis), almost always rash, and lymphadenopathy. Rheumatoid factors, antinuclear factors, and HLA-B27 are negative. Leukocytosis and anemia are common during active disease phases.
2. Seronegative polyarthritis. This occurs throughout childhood with no age peak. Rheumatoid factors and HLA-B27 are negative. Antinuclear factors are detectable in one of four cases.
3. Seropositive polyarthritis. Onset is usually after the age of ten. Girls are several times more likely to be affected than boys. HLA-B27 and rheumatoid factors are positive in all cases and antinuclear factors in 75% of cases. The disease frequently develops into the adult form of rheumatoid arthritis.
4. Type I (iridocyclitis type) oligoarthritis. Early onset before the age of six. The disease is several times more likely to affect girls than boys. Asymmetric involvement of large joints with chronic iridocyclitis in 50% of cases. Antinuclear factors are also present in 50% of cases (rheumatoid factors and HLA-B27 being negative).
5. Type II (sacroiliitis type) oligoarthritis. Onset is at school age, and 90% of those affected are boys. Asymmetric involvement of large joints.

Iridocyclitis is rare. By contrast, sacroiliitis is common. The disease can develop into ankylosing spondylitis.

Like rheumatoid arthritis in adults, juvenile polyarthritis is usually episodic in nature. The prognosis is far more favorable in oligoarticular forms than in polyarthritis.

Diagnosis and differential diagnosis. As in rheumatoid arthritis in adults, the diagnosis is based on the patient's history and the clinical picture (morning stiffness, swollen hot joints, possibly fever and pain), laboratory findings (elevated ESR and CRP, anemia, possibly rheumatoid factors, possibly antinuclear factors), and radiologic findings (periarticular swelling, periarticular osteoporosis, in the further course bone lesions, narrowing of the articular cavity, later deviation and subluxation). Table 5.**3** lists important differential diagnostic considerations.

Drug treatment. In JCA, too, effective drug treatment must be initiated as early as possible in parallel with nonpharmacologic measures in order to prevent irreversible sequelae such as joint destruction, visual disturbances secondary to iridocyclitis, growth disturbances, and organ failure (especially of the kidneys and intestines due to amyloidosis). Accordingly, the therapy must be adapted to the individual situation (subtype, disease stage, activity, age, psychosocial situation). Initiating and changing treatment is the purview of the specialist (pediatric rheumatologist). It is also the specialist who undertakes additional follow-up examinations at long intervals and is consulted if problems arise.

- All children receive a fast-acting **NSAID.** The dose is related to body weight. Drugs such as diclofenac (2–3 mg/kg 2–3 times daily), ibuprofen (10–20 mg/kg 3–4 times daily), indomethacin (2–3 mg/kg 3–4 times daily), or naproxen (10–15 mg/kg twice daily) are preferred to acetylsalicylic acid (50–80 mg/kg 3–4 times daily).
- **SAARDs** should be used early, especially in active polyarthritis and/or arthrodestructive forms as well as in Chauffard-Still syndrome:
  - In *type I oligoarthritis* an **antimalarial substance** is the drug of first choice (not if convulsions are likely – an EEG and history being mandatory). In the case of iridocyclitis which does not respond to local corticosteroid therapy, azathioprine or cyclosporin A should be given.
  - In *type II oligoarthritis* **sulfasalazine** is usually given. Azathioprine (possibly in combination with immunosuppressants), methotrexate, and cyclosporin are also suitable.
  - For the treatment of *seronegative and seropositive polyarthritis* the entire spectrum of conventional SAARDs can be considered. In mild cases or in combination with other SAARDs, one can initially resort to **chloroquine** or **hydroxychloroquine.**
  - In benign forms of Chauffard-Still syndrome an **antimalarial drug** is possible, otherwise azathioprine, methotrexate, or cyclosporin are indicated. Sulfasalazine, gold, and D-penicillamine are contraindicated in systemic JCA as they can trigger severe complications with disseminated intravascular coagulation.
  - *Amyloidosis* tends to occur mainly in Chauffard-Still syndrome but is treated in all subgroups with **chlorambucil.**
- In the nonsystemic forms of JCA **glucocorticoids** should be used with the utmost reservation.
  - In iridocyclitis local corticosteroid therapy and in rheumatic myocarditis systemic corticosteroid therapy is essential.
  - The intra-articular administration of triamcinolone may also be beneficial.
  - In connection with long-term corticosteroid therapy for systemic JCA, the dose should be

Table 5.**3** Differential diagnosis of juvenile chronic arthritis (selection)

- Juvenile ankylosing spondylitis
- Wissler's syndrome (subsepsis hyperergica) (must be diagnostically differentiated from Still-Chauffard syndrome!)
- Reactive (postinfectious) arthritides
- Rheumatic fever
- Infectious arthritides (TBC, Lyme borreliosis, viral diseases, mycoses)
- Systemic vasculitis (Behçet's syndrome, Kawasaki disease, infantile polyarteritis, etc.)
- Juvenile forms of collagen disease
- Leukoses, histiocytosis
- Sickle cell anemia, hemophilia
- Sarcoidosis
- Arthritis associated with mucoviscidosis, diabetic chiropathy, storage diseases, etc.
- Non-inflammatory bone diseases (trauma, aseptic bone necrosis, osteochondrosis dissecans, epiphysiolysis captis, osteoid osteoma, etc.)

kept low in children owing to the specific risk of side effects (maximum 0.15 mg/kg prednisolone equivalent daily) and should be given in single doses in the morning or in alternation.
- In highly active forms or in refractory iridocyclitis a three-day regimen of corticosteroid shock therapy with ultrahigh doses (10 – 20 mg/kg) has proven beneficial.

About four to six months after clinical and humoral abatement of the disease, the drug therapy is gradually reduced and finally withdrawn altogether.

5.4 Ankylosing spondylitis

Table 5.**4** Common features of spondylarthritides

- Arthritis with asymmetric joint involvement, usually oligoarticular and of the lower extremities
- Insertion tendopathies
- Dactylitis
- Sacroiliitis and other inflammations of the axial skeleton
- Typical extra-articular manifestations (uveitis, iridocyclitis, conjunctivitis, mucocutaneous lesions such as recurrent aphthous stomatitis, urethritis, psoriasiform skin lesions, erythema nodosa, etc.)
- Absence of rheumatoid factors and rheumatoid nodules
- Familial clustering and association with HLA-B27

Disease features. Ankylosing spondylitis (synonym Bekhterev's disease) is the prototype of a large group of seronegative spondylarthritides, which also includes diseases such as psoriatic arthritis, arthritis associated with Crohn's disease and ulcerative colitis, and B27-associated reactive arthritides with or without Reiter's syndrome (Table 5.**4**). In 80 – 90% of cases ankylosing spondylitis affects men with the incidence clearly peaking in the third decade of life. It is a chronic systemic inflammatory rheumatic disease associated with proliferative and destructive processes in the iliosacral and vertebral joints leading to gradual bony stiffening of the spine and kyphosis. The disease is episodic, and both painful and relatively painfree forms exist. In 50 – 70% of cases remittent or chronic extravertebral arthritis occurs. Characteristic of ankylosing spondylitis is a tendency towards insertion tendopathies. The most common organ manifestation is recurrent iritis or iridocyclitis. More rarely there is kidney involvement (amyloidosis, interstitial nephritis, IgA nephropathy). Even rarer are cardiovascular manifestations (aortitis, AV conduction disturbances, pericarditis, and myocarditis).

Diagnosis and differential diagnosis. Based on the typical epidemiology, early ankylosing spondylitis must be suspected in any young man with unclear back pain or arthritic symptoms. It should be noted that the disease often appears as mono- or oligoarthritis of proximal and distal joints (especially of the lower extremities). Peripheral joint involvement is usually oligoarticular and asymmetric, though bilateral involvement of the shoulder and hip joints is common.

In the early stage the cardinal symptom is deep lower back pain at night, often accompanied by morning stiffness in the lumbar and/or thoracic spine and generalized symptoms such as weakness, malaise, and occasionally subfebrile temperatures. An additional diagnostic indicator may be pain in the heels as an expression of insertion tendopathy. Iritis rarely precedes the disease but often accompanies it recurrently. A clinically striking feature is pain on compression of the iliosacral joints, impaired mobility of the spine (Schober's sign reduced, finger-to-floor distance increased), and thoracic rigidity (reduced respiratory expansion).

The humoral parameters of inflammation (ESR, CRP) are only moderately elevated and are often normal. HLA-B27 is usually positive. Early radiologic symptoms include characteristic iliosacral arthritis with concurrent destructive and proliferative changes as well as syndesmophytes in the thoracolumbar junction. In the advanced stage the typical bamboo shape of the spine is encountered with complete bridging syndesmophytes.

Ankylosing spondylitis must be distinguished mainly from other inflammatory and degenerative disease of the spine and iliosacral joints. Notably, these include other spondylarthritides, infectious spondylitis, Paget's disease, hyperostosis triangularis ilii, and hyperosotica spondylitis (Forrestier's disease). If only peripheral joints are affected in the early stage, the entire spectrum of mono- and oligoarthritis forms must be considered.

Drug therapy. In view of the protean nature of the clinical picture, treatment is based on the individual signs and symptoms. In addition to physiotherapy, local and systemic administration of analgesic and anti-inflammatory drugs (sometimes also muscle relaxants) is usually unavoidable.

- Pain and inflammation of the spine and proximal and peripheral joints usually respond adequately to **NSAIDs.** If the pain is severe, sufficient doses must be given and possibly i.v. phenylbutazone for a short period. To treat nocturnal pain it is advisable to administer a long-acting NSAID or a delayed-release dosage form rectally or orally. However, the decision to initiate long-term therapy (e.g. with a long-acting drug such as piroxicam) should be made with caution, since the prognosis is influenced imperceptibly by NSAIDs.
- **Systemic glucocorticoids** should only be used in exceptional circumstances and only temporarily, i.e. in cases of several peripheral joint involvement, disease episodes that cannot otherwise be controlled, and severe extra-articular complications.
- **Local corticosteroid therapy** is sensible and effective in some situations, e.g painful insertion tendopathy and tendinitis (paratendinous injection) as well as in NSAID-resistant pain due to marked sacroiliitis (infra-articular).
- **Muscle relaxants** can be used temporarily for treating painful myotendinosis.
- Analgesics come into consideration as adjuvant medication if the patient's pain is not relieved by NSAIDs alone.
- The value of SAARDs in the treatment of ankylosing spondylitis is controversial. However, in the presence of high activity of the spinal process, an attempt at treatment with **sulfasalazine** is permitted. In active polyarthritis a **gold preparation** or **methotrexate** may also be used.
- Extra-articular organ manifestations (eyes, heart, kidneys) are treated by specialists according to established principles.

5.5 Psoriatic arthritis

Disease features. The prevalence of psoriasis in the population is about 5%, and one in five psoriasis patients develops arthritis which is usually rheumatoid-factor negative. The joint disease usually occurs within 1–2 years of manifestation of the skin disease, rarely concurrently with or before the onset of psoriasis. The incidence peaks between the ages of 30 and 45 years. Etiologically, the main factor is a genetic predisposition (close association with HLA-B27). To date no exogenous factors have been identified. The clinical picture of psoriatic arthritis is highly variable, ranging from predominant involvement of the axial skeleton, as in ankylosing spondylitis, to the classical form with a preponderance of arthritis of the interphalangeal joints of the toes and fingers and typical psoriatic nail changes (Table 5.**5**). The affected joints are distended by joint effusion and capsule swelling. The skin may be red and warm. The disease is episodic and is associated with a high mortality rate due to concomitant diseases (cardiovascular system, lungs, malignancies).

Diagnosis and differential diagnosis. In view of the absence of "positive" diagnostic criteria, psoriatic arthritis is diagnosis by exclusion. Every case of arthritis occurring in conjunction with ex-

Table 5.**5** Forms of psoriatic arthritis

Type	Clinical picture	Approx. incidence
"Classical" psoriatic arthritis	Characterized by arthritis of the distal interphalangeal joints and nail defects.	5–15%
Symmetric arthritis similar to rheumatoid arthritis	Bilateral symmetrical involvement of large and small joints.	15–20%
Oligoarticular arthritis	Asymmetric involvement of large and small joints; periostitis of small joints leads to "sausage fingers" and dactylitis.	50–70%
Ankylosing spondylitis	Involvement of sacroiliac and spinal joints (also asymmetric); often in conjunction with other types of peripheral joint involvement.	5–20%
Arthritis mutilans	Osteolysis of the phalangeal and metacarpal joints; spondylitis.	5%

isting psoriasis is considered to be psoriatic arthritis as long as the joint disease does not meet the criteria of another form of arthritis. Care is required in the search for skin efflorescences. Predilection sites are the extensor sides of the extremities, scalp, sacral region, nails, and external auditory meatus. However, less typical locations of psoriatic arthritis also occur (the palms, soles of the feet, anal fold, navel, axillary folds, submammary area). In cases without evident skin manifestations the diagnosis of psoriatic arthritis can also be made in an otherwise typical clinical picture if a first-degree relative has confirmed psoriasis.

A diagnostic indication is asymmetric, oligoarticular joint involvement, typically affecting the interphalangeal joints of a finger or toe (ray involvement, "sausage finger").

Distal-joint arthritis is often associated with characteristic psoriatic nail changes (pitting, dystrophy, lifting, furrowing of the nail). Another typical set of findings resembles ankylosing spondylitis with involvement of sacroiliac and intervertebral joints as well as paravertebral ligaments. Here too the involvement may be asymmetrical. Patients often report typical deep low-back pain at night.

The laboratory findings are unspecific and the parameters of inflammation less marked than in rheumatoid arthritis. Rheumatoid factors are usually negative and the ESR is slightly to moderately accelerated. In cases of pronounced psoriatic efflorescences uric acid levels may be increased.

Radiologic examination reveals a clustering of destructive (bone defects) and proliferative (protuberances, periosteal reactions, fibrositis) changes of the joints, often with marked mutilations. Periarticular osteoporosis is absent.

The most common extra-articular manifestations of psoriatic arthritis are insertion tendopathies (e.g. of the heels and major trochanter), tenosynovitis, and manubriosternal synchondritis. Visceral involvement (iritis, amyloidosis, very rarely myositis) is rare.

Psoriatic arthritis with early mono- and oligoarticular involvement must be differentiated from reactive arthritides and other seronegative spondylarthritides, acute monoarthritis, and gout; in the case of polyarticular involvement from seronegative rheumatoid arthritis; in the case of psoriatic spondylitis from idiopathic ankylosing spondylitis.

Drug therapy. Therapy is fundamentally similar to treatment for rheumatoid arthritis or ankylosing spondylitis. However, the regimen must be adapted to the individual course of the disease. In addition, it must be borne in mind that some drugs can exacerbate the skin changes.

- **NSAIDs** are the drugs of first choice for arthritis and for joint and back pain. An adverse effect on the skin efflorescences is rare.
- The use of **SAARDs** is indicated in progressive cases that do not respond satisfactorily to NSAIDs. Experience in this context has been gained mostly with sulfasalazine and methotrexate.
  - **Methotrexate** in a dose of up to 25 mg daily induces an improvement of arthritic and skin symptoms in most patients. Parenteral use is also possible.
  - **Sulfasalazine** in a dose of 2 g daily leads to improvement of articular and serologic inflammatory activity. Skin manifestations are rarely exacerbated.
  - **Cyclosporin** is regarded as a reserve drug for refractory cases. The initial dose of 2.5–3 mg/kg daily can be increased up to 5 mg/kg daily. The skin symptoms usually improve first, followed with some delay by improvement of the joint symptoms.
  - Treatment with oral **auranofin** or i.m. **aurothiomalate** can be attempted, although the efficacy of this therapy is supported only by a small number of studies [Lacaille et al., 2000; Bruckle et al., 1994].
  - Chloroquine and hydroxychloroquine should not be used owing to the risk of dermatologic side effects.
- The intra-articular administration of **glucocorticoids** is also a highly effective treatment in mono- and oligoarticular psoriatic arthritis with a minimal potential for adverse effects.
- **Systemic corticosteroids** are often the last resort in highly active and refractory cases. Although they usually lead to improvement, reducing their dose or withdrawing them can lead to exacerbation of skin manifestations.
- The decision to use **systemic psoriasis drugs** should be made by a dermatologist.

5.6 Reactive arthritides

Disease features. The term reactive arthritis is applied to aseptic arthritis that develops over a period of few days to weeks (usually within 1–2 weeks) following an extra-articular, usually urogenital or gastrointestinal infection. The arthritis mainly affects the major joints of the lower extremities asymmetrically. Reiter's syndrome is a special form of reactive arthritis with additional urethritis and conjunctivitis (symptom triad) and sometimes skin changes (symptom tetrad). In addition, dactylitis ("sausage" fingers and toes), insertion tendopathy, and acute iliosacral arthritis may occur. Reactive arthritis disappears within a space of several months in 80 to 90% of cases. Occasionally, however, it can develop into chronic arthritis, sometimes with inflammatory involvement of the spine. This occurs particularly often in HLA-B27-positive male patients.

The causative agent in the urogenital tract is usually *Chlamydia trachomatis,* more rarely *Ureaplasma urealyticum,* in the gastrointestinal tract group B, C, and D salmonellae, shigellae, *Yersinia* spp., and *Campylobacter jejuni.* Live organisms have not been isolated from joints. However, with the help of sensitive methods researchers have discovered antigenic bacterial components which may trigger the arthritis via immunologic mechanisms.

Diagnosis and differential diagnosis. The diagnosis is based on inclusion and exclusion criteria (Table 5.**6**). If the history of infection is unclear, reactive arthritis needs to be differentiated from a number of diseases with similar joint involvement: ankylosing spondylitis with peripheral joint involvement, psoriatic arthritis, enteropathic arthritis (Crohn's disease, ulcerative colitis), Whipple's disease, Behçet's syndrome, Lyme disease, acute sarcoidosis (Löfgren's syndrome), septic arthritis, crystal-induced arthritis (gout, chondrocalcinosis), and atypical onset of rheumatoid arthritis.

Drug therapy. The prognosis for reactive arthritis is more favorable than for other inflammatory rheumatic diseases. However, although spontaneous remission occurs in most cases within an average period of 9–12 months, the possibility of chronification must also be considered when planning treatment.

- Treatment consists primarily of **NSAIDs.** The medication must be given continuously in sufficiently high doses. If necessary, analgesics may additionally be given.

Table 5.**6** Diagnostic and exclusion criteria for reactive arthritis [after Kingsley & Sieper, 1996]

Diagnostic criteria

- Typical arthritis (most likely to affect lower extremities, asymmetric oligoarthritis)
- Prior infection
- If clinically manifest diarrhea or urethritis occurred in the past 4 weeks, laboratory identification is desirable but not obligatory.
- If no clinically manifest infection occurred, laboratory identification is obligatory (direct identification of causative microorganism at the site of infection, e.g. by urethral or vaginal swab; indirect identification by increased titer of specific antibodies; demonstration of microbial components by means of the polymerase chain reaction or specific monoclonal antibodies).

Exclusion criteria

- Other known causes of mono- or oligoarthritis, e.g. confirmed ankylosing spondylitis, septic arthritis, Lyme disease, or reactive arthritis due to streptococci infection.
- Identification of HLA-B27, extra-articular manifestations of Reiter's syndrome, or typical features of spondylitides are not required for the diagnosis of reactive arthritis.

- The demonstration of chlamydiae in the urogenital tract requires adequate **antibiotic therapy** (including treatment of the patient's partner), e.g. with doxycycline (100 mg b.i.d.), ciprofloxacin (500 mg b.i.d.), ofloxacin (200 mg b.i.d.) or erythromycin (500 mg q.i.d.) over 10–14 days. In the case of gastroenteritis a 14-day course of fluoroquinolone is recommended, if streptococci are detected in a throat swab a ten-day course of penicillin (1 million units q.i.d.). Although the antibiotic treatment has no effect on the current arthritis, it can prevent later recurrences.
- **Systemic corticosteroid therapy** (0.2 to 1.5 mg prednisolone equivalent per kg body weight depending on the severity) is indicated for severe extra-articular manifestations, highly active polyarthritis, or fever.
- If no improvement occurs within three months, the use of an SAARD should be considered. **Sulfasalazine** mainly comes into consideration for this purpose.
- In *acute rheumatic fever* with severe carditis **corticosteroids** (1 mg prednisolone equivalent per kg body weight) should be used in-

stead of NSAIDs. For antibiotic therapy **benzylpenicillin** (1 million units daily once or twice daily) for ten days, alternatively also clemizole penicillin (1 million units once daily i.m.) or erythromycin (20–25 mg/kg daily) should be used. This is followed by **antibiotic recurrence prophylaxis.**

5.7 Systemic lupus erythematosus

Disease features. Systemic lupus erythematosus (SLE) is a chronic recurrent and remittent systemic inflammatory disease. The annual incidence in the USA is estimated to be 50–70 cases per million inhabitants and the prevalence 50 cases per 100,000. About 90% of those affected are female. The onset of the disease peaks between the ages of 20 and 40 years. For a hitherto unknown cause and favored by certain genetic characteristics, SLE patients develop reactive antibodies (autoantibodies) to endogenous cytoplasmic and nuclear antigens. The resulting antigen-antibody complexes accumulate in various organs, where they induce inflammatory reactions. The clinical picture is extremely varied and can also change in the course of the disease ("chameleon" character). The parts most often affected are the skin, joints, kidneys, nervous system, and serous membranes (pleura, pericardium). In addition, however, a number of other organs may also be affected. During active disease phases subfebrile temperatures or febrile episodes may occur. The patient loses weight and complains of tiredness, general malaise, and loss of appetite.

Diagnosis and differential diagnosis. Full-fledged SLE can be diagnosed in a straightforward manner with the help of the 1982 ARA criteria (Table 5.**7**). The diagnosis is confirmed if at least four criteria are met simultaneously or consecutively. In the early stage of the disease, however, the symptoms are often not fully developed, and the diagnosis is only made later in the course of the disease. Differential diagnostic possibilities include rheumatoid arthritis, other collagen diseases, hematologic systemic diseases, drug-induced SLE and pseudolupus erythematosus, (septic) infections, and in negative-ANA cases a complement defect syndrome.

Drug therapy. Not every case of SLE requires treatment. The therapeutic strategy is based on the current clinical findings and the progress of the disease and should not be based solely on serologic anomalies. The benefit of a therapeutic measure should always be weighed against the risk of adverse drug effects.

- Following the diagnosis of SLE all drugs that are known to be able to trigger such a disease or exacerbate the symptoms should be withdrawn and avoided. Notably, these include: hydralazine, procaine, hydantoin, oral contraceptives, allopurinol, and certain SAARDs (gold, D-penicillamine, sulfasalazine). The use of NSAIDs in SLE is associated with an increased risk of hypersensitivity reactions and dermatologic side effects [Ostensen und Villiger, 2001], warranting a reserved attitude and special caution. In particular, an increased incidence of meningitis and a negative effect on the disease symptoms have been reported for ibuprofen [Skaer, 1992; Jolles et al., 2000], which should therefore not be used.

Table 5.**7** 1982 diagnostic criteria of the American Rheumatism Association (ARA) for systemic lupus erythematosus

- Butterfly rash
- Discoid rash
- Increased photosensitivity (unusual skin reactions)
- Painless oral or nasopharyngeal ulceration
- Nonerosive arthritis involving at least two peripheral joints characterized by stiffness, swelling or effusion
- Pleurisy or pericarditis
- Renal disorder with persistent proteinuria > 0.5 g/day or cellular casts of erythrocytes, hemoglobin, tubular, granular or mixed
- Neurologic symptoms (seizures in the absence of other causes, psychoses)
- Hematologic findings (hemolytic anemia with reticulocytosis or leukopenia < 4000/µL or lymphopenia < 1500/µL or thrombocytopenia < 100 000/µL)
- Immunologic findings (LE cells or anti-DNA antibody or anti-Sm antibody or false-positive serologic for syphilis* for at least six months, confirmed by Treponema
- pallidum immobilization or fluorescent treponemal antibody)
- Antinuclear antibody (ANA titer > 1 : 160 in the immunofluorescence test)

* Due to phospholipid antibodies; nowadays these can be detected with high sensitivity by means of ELISA.

Depending on the severity of the case, certain NSAIDs, antimalarial drugs, corticosteroids, and, in severe cases, immunosuppressants are used.

- **NSAIDs** (not ibuprofen!) are used in severe musculoskeletal pain, serositis and headache.
- **Glucocorticoids** form a key element in the treatment of SLE. In acute and exacerbated cases the treatment is initiated with approximately 1 mg/kg daily prednisolone equivalent. Within 2–3 months an attempt should be made to reduce the corticosteroid to a lower maintenance dose or to end the therapy.
- In especially severe cases and life-threatening situations **shock therapy** with 500–1000 mg prednisolone i.v. for 3–5 days has proved beneficial.
- If treatment with NSAIDs and/or low-dose corticosteroids is insufficient, long-term treatment with **chloroquine** (max. 4 mg/kg daily) or **hydroxychloroquine** (max. 6.5 mg/kg daily) is an option for improving arthralgia and skin lesions or reducing the frequency of episodes.
- If the above measures prove insufficient and organ manifestations are threatening, the immunosuppressant **azathioprine** can be given in addition to corticosteroids and/or an antimalarial drug, e.g. in an initial dose of 2–2.5 mg/kg daily.
  - If improvement occurs, the corticosteroid should first be withdrawn gradually, followed by azathioprine, and finally the antimalarial drug.
- If inflammatory activity remains at a high level or if severe visceral manifestations (lupus nephritis, CNS manifestations) or vasculitis develop, **cyclophosphamide** is indicated, e.g. shock therapy with 500–1000 mg/m^2 every 3–4 weeks, once remission has been achieved every three months, for at least two years.
- In the presence of high antiphospholipid antibody titers **acetylsalicylic acid** (100 mg daily) should be given prophylactically to prevent thrombotic complications. Following a venous thrombotic event, **warfarin therapy** is indicated. The same applies for the treatment of recurrent arterial occlusions despite acetylsalicylic acid therapy.

5.8 Progressive systemic sclerosis

Disease features. Progressive systemic sclerosis is an inflammatory systemic connective-tissue disease characterized by thickening and hardening of the skin (scleroderma) and manifestations in other organ systems, including the vascular system, musculoskeletal system, gastrointestinal tract, lungs, heart, and kidneys. Its spontaneous course is extraordinarily variable and by no means always progressive. Women are affected three times more frequently than men, and the onset of the disease peaks after the age of 60. The etiology is unknown, although a clinical picture resembling scleroderma has been experimentally induced by various substances (vinyl chloride and other organic hydrocarbons, quartz dust, silicon, and the cytostatic bleomycin). A striking histologic finding is the deposition of connective-tissue substances (collagen, glycosaminoglycans) in the skin, vascular walls, and internal organs.

Diagnosis and differential diagnosis. The ARA criteria (Table 5.**8**) relate to pathognomic skin lesions which, however, only become clearly developed in the further course of the disease, giving the patient the sensation of skin that is too tight. An early – often the first – symptom is Raynaud's phenomenon, which should always raise the suspicion of scleroderma. The detection of antinuclear antibodies typical of scleroderma (positive in over 90% of cases) and typical capillary microscopic nailfold changes can lend support to the suspected diagnosis. Patients may also develop pulmonary functional disturbances with exertional dyspnea and cough, esophageal motility disturbance (dysphagia), and joint symptoms (pain, swelling, stiffness, crepitations) in an early stage. Involvement of the gastrointestinal tract is

Table 5.**8** 1980 scleroderma criteria of the American Rheumatism Association (ARA). The diagnosis is confirmed if the main criterion or two secondary criteria are met

Main criterion

- Scleroderma proximal to the metacarpophalangeal joints

Secondary criteria

- Sclerodactyly
- Pitting scars or substance loss from distal soft tissue of the fingers
- Bilateral basal fibrosis of the lungs

manifested as diarrhea and cramps. Among the less common disease manifestations are myopathy, pericarditis and heart failure, renal impairment, Sjögren's syndrome, and hypothyroidism.

Conditions to be ruled out by differential diagnosis are generalized forms of local scleroderma (morphea), Shulman's syndrome (eosinophilic fasciitis) scleroderma-like diseases induced by chemicals and environmental toxins, other collagen diseases, and mixed connective-tissue disease.

Drug therapy. Treatment of systemic sclerosis is difficult and often unsatisfactory. The therapeutic strategy concentrates on inhibiting inflammation by suppressing pathologic immune processes, preventing fibrosis, and improving the microcirculation. However, for many drugs no efficacy results are available from controlled studies. Treatment depends on the extent of skin and organ involvement.

In the *limited disease form,* which is largely restricted to peripheral parts and in which no vital organs are involved, treatment concentrates on **improving the microcirculation.** The patient should avoid nicotine as well as drugs containing clonidine and ergotamine. Stress and cold prophylaxis (warm clothing, gloves) is also important, and physical measures are beneficial. Medicinally, the following alternatives come into consideration:

- Long-term therapy with a **calcium antagonist,** e.g. nifedipine 20 – 30 mg daily.
- **Prostaglandin analogs,** e.g. infusions of carboprostacylin (Iloprost®) 2 ng/kg/min over 6 – 8 hours on 3 – 5 consecutive days or alprostadil (Prostavasin®) 60 µg over 3 hours for 10 – 14 days.
- **Pentoxifylline** (Trental®) 400 – 1200 mg daily.
- **Calcitonin** i. v. 100 IU for 10 days.
- Alpha receptor blockers such as **prazosin** (gradual dose introduction with escalation up to 4 – 5 mg daily).
- **Glucocorticoids** (initial dose 20 – 30 mg daily) are indicated only in the early edematous stage of the disease or in NSAID-refractory arthralgia. Long-term therapy should be avoided.

An attempt at treatment with immunosuppressants is indicated in *diffuse forms* of systemic sclerosis characterized by rapid progression and involvement of vital organs. Use of vasoactive drugs for the treatment of Raynaud's phenomenon also makes sense in this disease form.

- In active inflammatory lung involvement **cyclophosphamide** can bring about an improvement of pulmonary function (1 – 2.5 mg/kg daily in combination with low-dose **prednisolone** therapy).
- In various studies **methotrexate** (7.5 – 20 mg/week) led to improvement of the skin manifestations; in the early diffuse stage and in higher doses (25 – 50 mg/week) the drug prevented the development of further organ manifestations.
- **Azathioprine** (2 mg/kg daily) and **cyclosporin** (2.5 – 5 mg/kg) may also have a beneficial effect on the cutaneous manifestations. However, cyclosporin is associated with an increased risk of renal complications (malignant hypertension, renal impairment).
- Regression of skin thickening, a reduction in the number of new renal manifestations, improvement of pulmonary function, and prolongation of life expectancy have been observed in numerous uncontrolled studies with **D-penicillamine.** Disadvantages are a high rate of sometimes serious adverse effects (up to 20% of patients do not tolerate the drug) and a long drug latency period of around one year. Use of D-penicillamine should therefore remain limited to early diffuse diseases. Initial dose 250 mg daily, increased every two months up to a maintenance dose of 750 mg daily and, after the onset of the therapeutic effect, reduction if possible to 250 mg daily.
- In cases of high inflammatory activity, alveolitis, serositis, myositis, and in overlap syndrome (presence of characteristic symptoms of various collagen diseases) the additional administration of **glucocorticoids** is often unavoidable (prednisolone in an initial dose of 30 mg daily, increased to a maximum dose of 1 mg/kg daily). Caution: High-dose corticosteroids (≥ 15 mg prednisolone equivalent daily) can precipitate a renal crisis [Steen and Medsger, 1998].

5.9 Polymyositis and dermatomyositis

Disease features. Polymyositis and dermatomyositis are the best-known representatives of the idiopathic myositides. They are rare inflammatory diseases of the skeletal musculature which can occur isolated as well as in association with related collagen diseases or malignant tumors. Women are affected 2 – 3 times more often then men with the incidence peaking between the ages of 45 and 60. Clinically both diseases usually manifest themselves in stiffness-like muscle pain and myasthenia, especially of proximal muscles of the shoulder and pelvic girdles (difficulty standing up and lying down, climbing stairs, and lifting the arms. Later in the course of the disease the muscle weakness spreads distally. Often (nonerosive) polyarthritis with arthralgia is present. In addition, lung (pulmonary fibrosis, alveolitis) and heart (arrhythmia, conduction disturbances, cardiomyopathy) manifestations occur. Raynaud's phenomenon is also common. In addition, dermatomyositis is associated with numerous characteristic skin findings (reddish livid discoloration of the eyelids; partly squamous rash on finger and toe joints, knees, elbows, and ankle joints, telangiectases, etc.). The skin changes in the facial area together with mimic rigidity result in the appearance of myopathic face.

Diagnosis and differential diagnosis. The diagnosis is based on typical clinical findings. It is confirmed by the results of a muscle biopsy (characteristic myositis findings with inflammatory infiltrates, muscle-fiber necrosis with simultaneous signs of regeneration, atrophy, in the advanced stage fibrosis), by laboratory findings (elevated creatine kinase (not obligatory!) or other muscle enzymes, myositis-specific antibodies, during episodes also creatinuria and myoglobinuria), as well as an EMG. Inflammatory changes in the muscles can be seen by MRI, even if the laboratory findings are still normal.

The range of differential diagnoses includes secondary myositides associated with other collagen diseases as well as infectious, parainfectious, paraneoplastic, and drug-induced myositides.

Drug therapy. Treatment is symptom-oriented and relies essentially on corticosteroids and immunosuppressants.

- During episodes high-dose **glucocorticoid** therapy is indicated (initially 1 mg/kg prednisolone, after two weeks incremental reduction to the lowest possible maintenance dose; in severe cases possible initiation of three-day shock therapy).
- In corticosteroid-resistant cases **methotrexate** can be additionally given (10 – 15 mg weekly i. v., if required 40 mg weekly for 4 – 6 weeks). **Azathioprine** (2 mg/kg daily) is an alternative, if vasculitis is present also **cyclophosphamide.**
- **Cyclosporin** appears to be particularly effective in overlap syndrome (initial dose 3 mg/kg daily with gradual escalation while monitoring renal function and blood pressure). Onset of action approximately 6 – 8 weeks.
- Although interval therapy with **i.v. immune globulin** (1 – 2 g/kg/month) is expensive, it is effective and usually well tolerated and should be offered at least to young patients for a certain period.

5.10 Polyarteritis nodosa (PAN)

Disease features. Polyarteritis nodosa (PAN; synonym: panarteritis nodosa) is a rare necrotizing vasculitis of small and medium-sized arteries that predominantly affects middle-age and elderly men. Gross histologic examination reveals inflammatory infiltrates and fibrinoid deposits in the vascular wall. Clinically the disease ranges from mild, transient forms with a gradual onset to fulminant, progressive, rapidly fatal forms. In addition to general symptoms such as fever, anorexia, and weight loss, other manifestations include multiple organ involvement with nephritis, peripheral neuropathy, skin lesions, asymmetric polyarthralgia or arthritis, cardiomyopathy, and epididymitis, rarely involvement of the CNS, lungs, and eyes.

In etiopathogenic terms, two forms can be distinguished, which are also treated differently. The first is associated with hepatitis B or C and is regarded as an immune-complex vasculitis (with evidence of hepatitis antigens in the vascular wall). In the second form there is no proven link with a viral infection.

Diagnosis and differential diagnosis. There are currently two rival classification systems for PAN: the 1990 classification of the American College of Rheumatology (ACR) [Lightfoot et al., 1990] and a newer classification issued at the 1992 Chapel Hill Consensus Conference [Jennette et al., 1994]. The latter defines classical polyarteritis nodosa as vasculitis of small and medium-sized arteries *without* involvement of capillaries. Thus, the diagnosis is ruled out by the presence of glomerulonephritis. Diseases that only affect small and microscopic vessels, including glomerular and alveolar capillaries, fall into the category of microscopic angiitis.

According to the ACR classification (Table 5.9), at least three of ten criteria must be met for the diagnosis of PAN. In view of the variable clinical

Table 5.**9** Classification of the American College of Rheumatology for polyarteritis nodosa [Lightfoot et al., 1990]

- Weight loss of more than 4 kg, general symptoms
- Livedo reticularis (extremities or trunk)
- Testicular tenderness and swelling
- Myalgia, weakness, tenderness of leg muscles
- Mono- or polyneuropathy, CNS syndrome
- Hypertension (diastolic blood pressure > 90 mm Hg)
- Serum creatinine > 1.5 mg/dL
- Detection of hepatitis B virus (surface antigens or antibodies)
- Arteriographic findings: aneurysms, occlusions
- Typical histologic changes of small and medium-sized arteries (evidence of granulocytes infiltrating the vascular wall ± mononuclear leukocytes)

picture of PAN, however, the practicality of this system is limited for individual diagnostic work. The laboratory findings are also uncharacteristic with a marked ESR increase, elevated CRP levels, leukocytosis, anemia, and slight eosinophilia. Rheumatoid factors and autoantibodies (ANCA, ANA) are rarely positive. A diagnostic indicator is provided by characteristic angiographic findings in the clinically affected organs, especially the liver, kidneys, and mesenteric arteries with aneurysms, stenoses, and sudden lumen changes. The diagnosis is confirmed by histologic findings of vascular wall changes. PAN must be differentiated from other vasculitides, collagen diseases, and systemic diseases.

Drug therapy. The poor prognosis of PAN has been significantly improved through the use of high-dose corticosteroids in conjunction with cytostatics. The therapeutic procedure depends largely on the extent and activity and on the pathogenesis of the disease, a distinction being be made between hepatitis-virus-associated (HBV or HCV) and non-hepatitis-associated disease.

Non-HBV or HCV-associated PAN

- Patients initially receive a **corticosteroid** in a starting dose of 1 – 2 mg/kg daily prednisolone equivalent (60 – 90 mg daily); if indicated, treatment may also be initiated with shock therapy. Once arteritic activity has subsided, the dose is gradually reduced to an effective maintenance dose.
- If the response to corticosteroid therapy is unsatisfactory, **cyclophosphamide** is additionally given; in severe forms, especially where there is renal and/or pulmonary involvement, combination therapy is indicated from the outset. Cyclophosphamide is administered according to the Fauci regimen (2 to max. 3 – 4 mg/kg daily p. o.).
- If full remission or at least stable partial remission has not been achieved after six to twelve months' treatment and low-dose prednisolone ((≤ 5 mg daily) is also required, the treatment can be changed to a less aggressive remission-maintaining regimen, e.g. **low-dose methotrexate** (only if renal function has been normalized) or **azathioprine.**

HBV- or HCV-associated PAN

- In organ- or life-threatening cases initial **immunosuppressive combination therapy** is also indicated in such cases. In addition, numerous small studies and case descriptions in recent years have reported good success with new therapeutic regimens that can also be used in less severe forms.
- In HBV-associated PAN a combination of **plasmapheresis** and **antiviral therapy,** e.g. with vidarabine or lamivudine, is indicated.
- In HCV-associated PAN **interferon alpha 2 a/2 b,** possibly in combination with **ribavirin;** the benefit of concurrent plasmapheresis in this regimen is still uncertain.

5.11 Gout and gouty arthritis

Disease features. Gout includes a range of disease manifestations, all of which are caused by hyperuricemia. Although the incidence of hyperuricemia in the population is extraordinarily high at 20 – 25 %, only about one in ten of those affected develop manifest gout. Several mechanisms can contribute to the accumulation of uric acid. In addition to a genetic disorder of purine metabolism, these include dietary factors, diseases associated with increased cell destruction, drug influences, and reduced renal excretion. When the solubility of uric acid in body fluids is exceeded, urate crystals precipitate in joints and periarticular structures (arthritis), soft tissue (tophi), the kidneys (gouty nephropathy), and the urinary tract (urate calculi). A typical gout attack is characterized by acute, extremely painful joint swelling and heat, bluish-red discoloration, edema, sometimes effusion, and generalized symptoms. Initially only a single joint is usually affected, most commonly the metatarsophalangeal joint of the great toe (podagra). Without treatment new gout attacks occur at ever shorter intervals, and after several years the condition progresses to the final stage of chronic gout with constant polyarticular arthritis, predominantly in the joints of the lower extremities. In addition, tophi occur in the bursae, auriculae, elbows, and Achilles' tendons. In many cases urate nephropathy is also present.

Diagnosis and differential diagnosis. Although the large majority of gout patients have hyperuricemia, this in itself is not a sufficient criterion for the diagnosis. The diagnosis is based instead on typical clinical features (podagra or at least two typical attacks in other joints followed by spontaneous remission). It is confirmed by the chemical or microscopic identification of urate crystals in synovial fluid or tissue. During an ongoing attack the differential diagnosis must consider pseudogout, (chondrocalcinosis), infectious arthritis, other arthritis forms accompanied by erythema, psoriatic arthritis, and bacterial infections (erysipelas, phlegmon) or thrombophlebitis. Chronic tophaceous gout must be differentiated from rheumatoid arthritis, psoriatic arthritis, and other deforming chronic arthritides.

Drug therapy. In acute gout attacks therapeutic efforts focus initially on eliminating the inflammatory symptoms. After the attack the objective is to control the metabolic disorder in the long term, avert recurrent attacks, and prevent complications. Asymptomatic hyperuricemia of up to 8 mg/dL does not require drug therapy.

- In acute gout attacks **NSAIDs** are the drugs of first choice. Drugs with a short half-life and rapid onset of action should be used, e.g. diclofenac (75 mg every six hours), indomethacin (25 – 50 mg every 4 – 6 hours) or phenylbutazone (possibly short term i.m.). Once the symptoms have improved, treatment is continued with 25 – 50 (max. 100) mg daily for at least three months.
- A specific (obsolete!) alternative drug for acute attacks is **colchicine,** which, however, acts more slowly than NSAIDs (prompt improvement of symptoms in response to colchicine can confirm the diagnosis of gout in etiologically unclear arthritis). Initially 1 mg is given, then 0.5 – 1 mg p.o. (maximum 8 mg) daily every two hours, with the dosage being reduced from day two. Colchicine can also be given in addition to NSAIDs (in which case the dose is 0.5 mg b.i.d.). Caution: Colchicine has a very narrow therapeutic window; an overdose is life-threatening!
- Only in severe refractory cases are **glucocorticoids** indicated (prednisolone 30 – 50 mg daily p.o., if large joints are affected possibly triamcinolone crystal suspension 40 mg intra-articularly) followed by further treatment with low-dose NSAID or colchicine.
- After an attack lifelong therapy with **uricosurics** or **uricostatics** is indicated in addition to dietary measures. Drugs of both classes should be introduced gradually and in the first few months should be combined with an NSAID so as not to provoke an attack. In cases of high urinary uric acid levels uricosuric drugs should not be used.
  - **Allopurinol,** which has a uricostatic effect is the drug of first choice (initially 100 – 200 mg daily, maintenance dose usually 200 – 300 mg daily). The daily dose can be taken at once.
  - Combination uricostatic-uricosuric therapy is possible and in tophaceous forms is sometimes also beneficial initially (e.g. **allopurinol** 100 mg daily and **benzbromarone** 20 mg daily).
- In urate nephropathy and nephrolithiasis **alkalization of the urine,** e.g. with Uralyt-U®, is indicated in addition to ensuring sufficient fluid intake (approximately 3 L per day).

5.12 Osteoarthritides

Disease features. The term osteoarthritis is applied to degenerative, primarily noninflammatory changes of the cartilaginous and bony structure of joints. Over the course of years it can lead to deformities of the joints with significant functional impairment. It mainly affects weight-bearing joints of the lower extremities (hip and knee joints and metatarsophalangeal joint of the great toe), more rarely the elbow, shoulder, hand, and finger joints. Osteoarthritis is so widespread as to be a commonplace disease. Its incidence rises significantly with age. Joint changes can be radiologically detected in 25% of 50-year-olds and in more than 80% of people over 80 years of age; the majority of those affected, however, remain

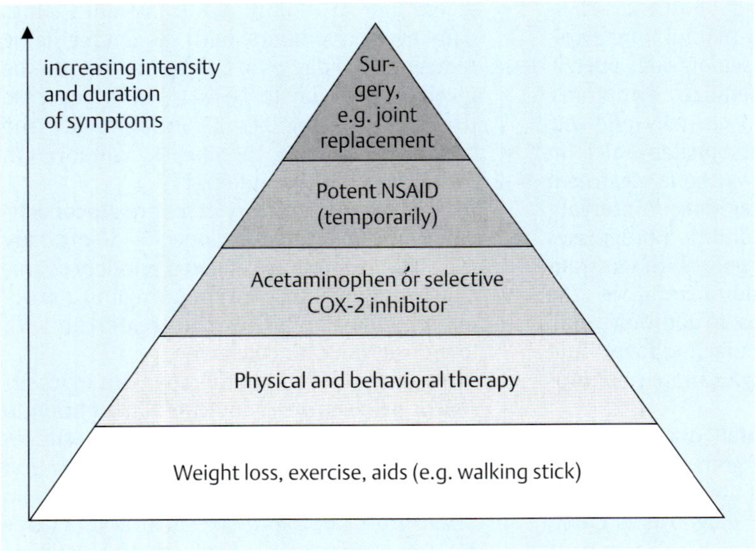

Fig. 5.**2** Treatment pyramid: procedure for treating active osteoarthritis.

asymptomatic (so-called silent or latent osteoarthritis). Sporadically, however, cartilage wear can lead to synovitis with its classical signs of inflammation; in this case the condition is referred to as active osteoarthritis. The result of progressive functional decompensation and joint destruction is continuous pain.

Diagnosis and differential diagnosis. The cardinal symptom is pain, which often has the character of initial pain on joint movement but worsens in the course of the day under stress. Only in the active stage does pain at rest and continuous pain occur. Heat and redness are absent except in the active stage. Joint swelling is firm, fluctuating only in active osteoarthritis with secondary synovitis (effusion). Sometimes crepitations are perceptible during functional tests of the joint. Since osteoarthritis is a local pathogenic process, systemic signs of inflammation are absent, in contrast to arthritis. Also, the ESR is at most slightly increased in active osteoarthritis. There is early radiologic evidence of narrowing of the articular cavity. Other characteristic changes are osteophytes, capsular ossification, subchondral bone thickening, and in the advanced stage cystoid spongiosal defects (ganglionic cysts).

Drug therapy. Treatment of painful osteoarthritis is oriented to the clinical picture, taking into consideration the patient's age, concurrent diseases, and lifestyle. The primary aims are to eliminate pain, improve mobility, and delay the disease's progression in the long term. Drug therapy plays an important role in the overall therapeutic concept, which includes general measures (weight loss, exercise), active physiotherapy, and surgery (Fig. 5.**2**).

It should be ensured that the osteoarthritic patient experiences pain relief without being exposed to or jeopardized by adverse drug effects.

- For the treatment of painful (decompensated) osteoarthritis without signs of inflammation **acetaminophen** (up to 4 g daily) clearly used to be the analgesic of first choice thanks to its low rate of side effects. Today a **selective cyclooxygenase (COX 2) inhibitor** (known as a coxib) can be used as an alternative (Table 5.**10**).
- If the symptoms are pronounced, and especially in active osteoarthritis, a potent **NSAID** can be given instead of acetaminophen or a coxib (Table 5.**10**). However, the treatment should be limited and adapted to the pain intensity (no pain prophylaxis!; use only as needed and in the required minimum dose!). In elderly patients drugs with a short half-life should be given preference, and renal function and the gastrointestinal tract should be monitored closely. **Note:** Coxibs are generally well tolerated. Gastrointestinal reactions are significantly less common than with classical NSAIDs. However, fluid retention and a usually mild and reversible elevation of blood pressure may occur, especially in elderly patients.

Table 5.**10** Properties and dosages of the most important analgesics and NSAIDs for the treatment of osteoarthritis

Pharmacokinetic, pharmacodynamic drug class	Oral bio-availability	Terminal elimination half-life ($t_{1/2}$)	Individual dose (maximum daily dose) in adults	Contraindications	(Typical) adverse effects (approx. incidence in %)	(Major) drug interactions
Low potency/rapid elimination/no COX-2 selectivity						
Acetaminophen (paracetamol)	70–90 %	2–4 h	0.5–1.5 g (4 g)	▪ Hypersensitivity ▪ Severe hepatic impairment	Rarely in therapeutic doses; after overdose: ▪ nausea, vomiting, drowsiness ▪ Hepatotoxicity ▪ Nephrotoxicity	▪ Alcohol, cytochrome P450 inducers: hepatotoxicity of acetaminophen ↑ (?)
Ibuprofen	100 %	2 h	200–800 mg (2.4 g)	▪ Effect on blood clotting ▪ reversible Hypersensitivity ▪ Pregnancy ▪ Ulcers	▪ Gastrointestinal ulcers[1] (dose > 1.2 g daily), bleeding (2–4 %) ▪ Analgesic asthma ▪ Analgesic headache, dizziness, tinnitus, loss of hearing ▪ Nephrotoxicity ▪ Reye's syndrome (?) (children with viral infection)	▪ Beta blockers: antihypertensive effect ↓ ▪ Lithium: lithium level ↑ ▪ loop/thiazide diuretics: antihypertensive and diuretic effect ↓ ▪ ACE inhibitors: effect ↓
Moderate potency/delayed elimination/no COX-2- selectivity						
Naproxen	90–100 %	12–15 h[3]	250–500 mg (1.25 mg)	Like ibuprofen	Like ibuprofen (dose effect smaller) ▪ Gastrointestinal effects ↑ ▪ Ototoxicity ↑ ▪ Edema[2] ↑	Like ibuprofen
High potency/rapid elimination/no COX-2 selectivity						
Diclofenac	~ 50 % dose-dependent	1–2 h[4]	25–75 mg (150 mg)	Like ibuprofen	Like naproxen, plus ▪ Nephro- and hepatotoxicity ↑	Like ibuprofen

continuation next page

Table 5.10 Properties and dosages of the most important analgesics and NSAIDs for the treatment of osteoarthritis

Pharmacokinetic, pharmacodynamic drug class	Oral bioavailability	Terminal elimination half-life ($t_{1/2}$)	Individual dose (maximum daily dose) in adults	Contraindications	(Typical) adverse effects (approx. incidence in %)	(Major) drug interactions
High potency/slow elimination/COX-2-selective activity						
Celecoxib	20–60% dose-dependent	9–11 h	100 mg (400 mg)	Like rofecoxib, plus sulfonamide allergy	Like rofecoxib	Like rofecoxib, plus: ▪ Fluconazole: celecoxib levels ↑ ▪ Lithium: lithium level ↑
Rofecoxib	~90	17 h	12.5 mg (25 mg)	▪ Hypersensitivity ▪ Analgesic asthma ▪ Hepatic/renal functional impairment	▪ Dyspepsia, diarrhea, abdominal pain (4–9%), ulcers, bleeding (< 0.1%) ▪ Elevated transaminase levels ▪ Nephrotoxicity ▪ Edema (~10%)	▪ ACE inhibitors: antihypertensive effect ↓ ▪ Rifampicin: rofecoxib level ↓ ▪ Methotrexate: MTX level ↑ ▪ Oral anticoagulants: INR ↑

1 Gastrointestinal bleeding/perforation after acidic nonselective COX inhibitors results in approx. 2000 deaths a year in Germany. In around 90% of cases patients > 60 years are affected. "Ulcer protection only be achieved with proton pump inhibitors, misoprostol (synthetic prostaglandin, leads to diarrhea and cramps) or nonacidic (selective) COX inhibitors. Glucocorticoids increase the risk of ulcers.

2 The incidence and intensity of water and electrolyte retention correlates with the potency and elimination half-life of the drug

3 Enterohepatic circulation.

Theoretically there is a risk of an increased incidence of thromboembolic diseases. *Patients with cardiovascular risks* should therefore be treated as follows:
- Acetaminophen + low-dose acetylsalicylic acid or
- NSAID + proton pump inhibitor + low-dose acetylsalicylic acid or
- Coxib + low-dose acetylsalicylic acid (indication not yet confirmed).

- If small joints are affected, e.g. osteoarthritis of finger joints, a **topical anti-inflammatory drug** can additionally be used (ibuprofen, felbinac, diclofenac, indomethacin); if larger joints are effected no therapeutic effect can be expected from topical application.
- In cases with high-grade inflammatory activity that cannot otherwise be controlled, an **intra-articular corticosteroid injection** can be considered, particularly if articular effusion is also present. In principle this procedure is contraindicated in nonactive osteoarthritis (cartilage necrosis!), especially in osteoarthritis of the hip (bone necrosis!). Also, no more than four injections should be administered per year (minimum interval between injections four weeks). The dosage of the drug (e.g. dexamethasone palmitate) depends on the size of the joint.
- Although so-called **chondroprotectants** (drugs that are claimed to have a cartilage-protecting or regenerating effect), e.g. chondroitin sulfate and hyaluronic acid, have exhibited positive effects in experiments and to some extent in clinical studies, scientific evidence does not yet warrant a general therapeutic recommendation. **Note:** The common practice of treating painful osteoarthritic joints by local injections of drugs is controversial. Injection of glucocorticoids may bring about temporary pain relief but can also cause further damage to degenerative osteoarthritic joints. The benefits of injecting hyaluronic acid and similar metabolic products of connective tissue have not been substantiated despite several publications. Experiments are currently underway in the USA to implant endogenous cartilage cells in osteoarthritic joints (after shaping the destroyed articular surfaces). Convincing, scientifically reproducible findings are still awaited.
- **Opioid analgesics** are not usually indicated in osteoarthritis. Only in exceptional cases can tramadol, for example, be used in elderly patients if NSAIDs are contraindicated, renal function is impaired, or other pain therapy proves inadequate.

5.13 References

Arnett FC, Edworthy SM, Bloch DA, et al. The American Rheumatism Association 1987 revised criteria for the classification of rheumatoid arthritis. Arthritis Rheum 1988; 31: 315 – 324

Bruckle W, Dexel T, Grasedyck K, Schattenkirchner M. Treatment of psoriatic arthritis with auranofin and gold sodium thiomalate. Clin Rheumatol 1994; 13: 209 – 216

Brune K, Krebs S, Manger B. Rheumatische Erkrankungen. In: Lemmer B, Brune K (Hrsg). Fülgraff Palm Pharmakotherapie. 11. Aufl. München: Urban & Fischer, 2001: 330 – 348

Jennette JC, Falk RJ, Andrassy K, et al. Nomenclature of systemic vasculitides. Proposal of an international consensus conference. Arthritis Rheum 1994; 37: 187 – 192

Jolles S, Sewell WA, Leighton C. Drug-induced aseptic meningitis: diagnosis and management. Drug Saf 2000; 22: 215 – 226

Kingsley G, Sieper J. Third International Workshop on Reactive Arthritis, 23 – 26 September, Berlin, Germany. Ann Rheum Dis 1996; 55: 564 – 570

Lacaille D, Stein HB, Raboud J, Klinkhoff AV. Longterm therapy of psoriatic arthritis: intramuscular gold or methotrexate? J Rheumatol 2000; 27: 1922 – 1927

Lightfoot RW, Michel BA, Bloch DA, et al. The American College of Rheumatology 1990 criteria for the classification of polyarteritis nodosa. Arthritis Rheum 1990; 33: 1088 – 1093

Ostensen M, Villiger PM. Nonsteroidal anti-inflammatory drugs in systemic lupus erythematosus. Lupus 2001; 10: 135 – 139

Skaer TL. Medication-induced systemic lupus erythematosus. Clin Ther 1992; 14: 496 – 506

Steen VD, Medsger TA. Case-control study of corticosteroids and other drugs that either precipitate or protect from the development of scleroderma renal crisis. Arthritis Rheum 1998; 41: 1613 – 1619

Abbreviations

AA	Arachidonic acid
ATLs	Aspirin-triggered lipoxins
cAMP	Cyclic adenosine monophosphate
BLT	Leukotriene B_4 receptor
BP	Blood Pressure
CNS	Central Nervous System
COX	Cyclooxygenase enzymes (e.g. COX-1 and COX-2)
CYP450	Cytochrome P450
CysLT	Cysteinyl-leukotriene receptors (e.g. CysLT1 and CysLT2)
DP	Prostaglandin D_2 receptor
ED_{50}	Effective concentration for 50% response
EETs	Epoxyeicosatrienoic acids
EP	Prostaglandin E_2 receptor
FLAP	5-lipoxygenase activating protein
FP	Prostaglandin F_2 receptor
GFR	Glomerular filtration rate
GM-CSF	Granulocyte-macrophage-colony-stimulating factor
GT	Gastrointestinal tract
HPETEs	Hydroperoxyeicosatetraenoic acids
HETEs	Monohydroxyeicosatetraenoic acids
IC_{50}	Concentration that reduces effect by 50%
ID_{50}	Dose that reduces effect by 50%
IL	Interleukin (e.g. IL-6, IL-1β, IL-10)
IFN	Interferon (e.g. IFN-α and IFN-β)
IP	Prostaglandin I_2 receptor
IP_3	Inositol phosphate
LTs	Leukotrienes (e.g. LTA_4, LTB_4, LTC_4, LTD_4, LTE_4)
LOX	Lipoxygenase (e.g. 5-LOX, 12-LOX and 15-LOX)
LPS	Lipopolysaccharide
LXs	Lipoxins (e.g. lipoxin A_4; lipoxin B_4)
mPGE	Microsomal prostaglandin E
Min	Multiple intestinal neoplasia gene
MPO	Myeloperoxidase
MN	Mononuclear cells
NF-κB	Nuclear factor kappa B
NK	Natural killer
NO	Nitric oxide
NSAIDs	Nonsteroidal anti-inflammatory dugs
OA	Osteoarthritis
OVLT	Organum vasculosum lamina terminalis (of the hypothalamus)
PAF	Platelet-activating factor
PGs	Prostaglandins (e.g. PGD_2, PGE_2, PGE_1, $PGF_{2\alpha}$, PGG_2, PGH_2)
PGDH	Prostaglandin dehydrogenase
PGHS	Prostaglandin H_2 synthase, prostaglandin endoperoxide synthase
PGI_2	Prostacyclin
PLA_2	Phospholipase A_2
$cPLA_2$	Cytosolic phospholipase A_2
$iPLA_2$	Calcium-independent phospholipase A_2
$sPLA_2$	Secretory phospholipase A_2
PMN	Polymorphonuclear leukocytes
p.o.	Orally (per os)
PPARs	Peroxisome proliferator-activated receptors
PUB	Upper gastrointestinal perforations, ulcers and bleeds
PUFA	Polyunsaturated fatty acids
RA	Rheumatoid arthritis
SRS-A	Slow-reacting substances of anaphylaxis
TGF	Transforming growth factor
TNF	Tumor necrosis factor
TP	Thromboxane A_2 receptor
TXs	Thromboxanes (e.g. thromboxane A_2 and thromboxane B_2)
UD_{50}	Ulcerogenic dose for 50% effect

Index

Page numbers in **bold** type refer to major entries.
Page numbers in *italic* type refer to figures or tables.

F

G

H

I